BRAINWRECK

A Healthcare Derailment

GAIL IRWIN

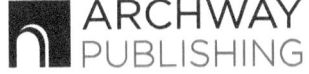

This book is a work of non-fiction. Unless otherwise noted, the author and the publisher make no explicit guarantees as to the accuracy of the information contained in this book and in some cases, names of people and places have been altered to protect their privacy.

Archway Publishing books may be ordered through booksellers or by contacting:

Archway Publishing
1663 Liberty Drive
Bloomington, IN 47403
www.archwaypublishing.com
844-669-3957

Because of the dynamic nature of the Internet, any web addresses or links contained in this book may have changed since publication and may no longer be valid. The views expressed in this work are solely those of the author and do not necessarily reflect the views of the publisher, and the publisher hereby disclaims any responsibility for them.

Any people depicted in stock imagery provided by Getty Images are models, and such images are being used for illustrative purposes only. Certain stock imagery © Getty Images.

Interior Image Credit: Angela Farinelli, ArtVista

ISBN: 978-1-6657-6753-8 (sc)
ISBN: 978-1-6657-6754-5 (e)

Library of Congress Control Number: 2024922099

Print information available on the last page.

Archway Publishing rev. date: 12/02/2024

DEDICATION
To my daughters Anne and Laura
For carrying my load when I could not
Forever grateful

THANKS TO
Serena Rinker
Extraordinary book assistant
Margaret Brabham, retired RN (1947-2023)
Medical record interpretation

SPECIAL MENTION
Royal Palm Beach Writers Group
Inspiration and elucidation

Contents

III. ASSISTED lIVING

IV. A STORIED TALE

Why Not Me?

My compact narrative, *Brainwreck*, bears a hefty wallop to awaken readers about inadequacies in our healthcare systems. Sound judgment and reasoning are at the core of good medical and post-medical care. If lacking, lives can be derailed, as was mine. And who better to write of this uncanny odyssey than myself. It is a cautionary tale. Others in like circumstances might plead "Why me?" I cannot. Instead, I chose to take a pivotal stance by dissecting, investigating, and analyzing conditions that left me critically ill following an emergency room visit after a fall to stitch up a head wound.

I grew up in a time when the medical credo was "The doctor knows best." Others my age did too. Now as elders, healthcare needs may become more prevalent and serious in nature. They may lead to a crisis. Yet, these crises can happen to anyone, anywhere, anytime. While medical science has greatly advanced over the years, even more so has the information age. Make knowledge your best weapon in handling healthcare decisions. Expert, reliable resource materials are available in every format. Seek them out. Use them. The day of leaving care solely to medical professionals and care facilities is over. Become a medical advocate for yourself and family members. The doctor may not always be right.

Brainwreck will catapult you through my own healthcare experiences from hospitalization to nursing home, then on to assisted living (AL). There are no falsehoods in my tale. Some events may astound and unnerve you but give valid testimony that strong personal oversight and advocacy are needed for hospital patients and care facility residents.

A hard fall outside my home resulting in a head laceration was the beginning of my tale. Twenty-six days after entry into a hospital emergency room for treatment, I was discharged, critically ill, to a nursing home. I had no major illnesses or minor ones when I entered the ER. How did this happen? The question lingered with me and my two daughters.

The huge sticking point came with my inability to remember anything of those hospital days. And yet, I wasn't sure if I even wanted to. Fabricated recollections made during hospitalization had cemented themselves into my mental space where real memories might have gone. Now, years later, I'd like to keep it that way. I feel it was a protective device. I have included several of my dreams throughout the book for readers to ponder about the curiosities of the mind.

After many months of nursing home care, I progressed to assisted living. I was still wheelchair bound. As I gained a smidgeon of strength each day, I finally felt it necessary to have a look at my medical records. Increasingly, I began to realize the big, bold question mark hanging over me of why I became so ill needed resolution. After a request to the hospital's record storage unit, a yardstick-high box of paperwork was delivered to my apartment door. Slowly, I sifted through it paring down the stack to a meaningful and manageable size. I kept the clinical records, the discharge report, exam findings, and surgery reports. This over one-foot-high heap of records would serve as my trail of enlightenment.

My fact-finding methodology was limited. Armed only with a medical dictionary, help from a Palm Beach County consumer librarian, and library Books-by-Mail, I began to dig in. I had no computer in my apartment, having had to relinquish most of my belongings when it became clear I'd never return home. Occasionally, I'd wheelchair over to the facility library hoping to do a little research. Often the computer was down, but that's facility life. To speed up record interpretation, I tried to find a local nurse or paralegal to help with specific explanations. No takers. I was tagged "it." The mission became one I pledged not to abandon, and the book slowly began to gel. Only later did I find a retired nurse I had known, now living out of state, to help review and explain medical record specifics.

I'm not going to apologize for the cliché, "Adding insult to injury," used by a friend when I related unruly and raucous, post-hospital events that had occurred in a large, corporate, assisted living facility. To evolve from a nappied (diapered), tube fed, wheelchair bound, extremely fatigued individual to a semi-independent human being, I needed a stress-free environment. Not one infused with its own detrimental company policy issues passed on to residents. Wellness shrinks from these surroundings. But I was surrounded and stuck.

Repeatedly, I've been told I should write a book. Now as a medically derailed octogenarian, I will oblige, hoping to swing readers from medical naivete to knowledge empowerment. It's hard for me to believe my experiences were one-of-a-kind. Yet they may have had a purpose. You become the judge. Is healthcare on the right track?

1

HOSPITALIZATION

Down But Not Out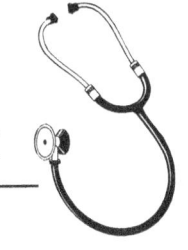

Each year, three million older people are treated in emergency rooms for fall injuries according to the Center for Disease Control and Prevention. In the year 2017, I was one of them sustaining a slip-per-fall injury, my pun for slip-and-fall. On this May 10 Sunday morning, the best newspaper day of the week, mine had not yet been delivered. I reported it to the Palm Beach Post. The newspaper is usually quick to respond, but not on this day. After waiting an hour or so and not hearing the paper hit my door, the usual signal, I went outside to look for it. Perhaps it was on the grass or behind my car in the two-vehicle driveway. Nowhere to be seen. Stepping forward on the concrete to return inside, my right foot propelled my slip-on slipper ahead without its occupant in it. Suspended in the air with no split-second message from foot to brain telling it what to do, I went off balance. Back went the right foot, then the left trying to compensate. Right, then left again gaining backwards momentum on the slightly sloped driveway. Reeling, down I went, backside on cement. My torso tried to break the fall, but an adult head is heavy and my skinny, non-muscular neck could not slow down the force of my head striking cement like an unleased bowling ball hitting the alley.

I may have been briefly stunned, but almost on cue the reality of "This is a fine mess you've gotten yourself into" kicked in. In my small, senior townhouse community, who would be out to notice me sprawled on the driveway on a Sunday morning. No one. I waited. Maybe a neighbor on the way to church would see me. Not going to happen. Yell, "Help!" Waste of energy.

My focus switched to getting back inside. I pulled myself into a babyish, pre-crawl position and slowly inched my way up the driveway. Scraping my arms and legs on the cement was more of a worry than what was going on in the back of my head. As I progressed to the door, blood was trickling down and leaving a trail behind me. I struggled to get up the porch and entryway step, then through the screen door. Still on all fours, my soft, comfortable recliner chair came into view. Ah! Just let me get there, get in the chair, and rest. I'd made it!

Still resting in the recliner, but not aware of time elapsed, my stomach was calling for a snack. I ventured into the kitchen. There was nothing snack worthy in the refrigerator. A bag of chips beckoned on the counter across from me. I took a few steps toward the counter to grab the bag. I felt woozy. The room began to spin, and down I went again. Nine-one-one time.

The telephone was not reachable from the floor. Wisely, I knew better than trying to get up again. The dangling phone cord caught my eye. Yes, I could possibly get hold of it, barely. Repeatedly, stretching and tugging at it, the phone fell within my grasp. I dialed.

Palm Beach County Fire Rescue was dispatched and on its way. When they arrived, I was alert and denied loss of consciousness, their report said. After reading Fire Rescue's report, which was included in the medical records I later obtained, I noted incomplete details making the writeup not entirely accurate. I called the rescue service to ask if there was a protocol used in gathering information. Were questions repeated or rephrased? Did they ask for more details or clarify medications? A proper diagnosis starts with the medic's report. I was told the team does what it feels is necessary and that it may vary depending on who is responding to the call.

Fire rescuers answered the report's descriptive captions as follows: Primary Impression – injury of head; Incident Type – fall with injury; Head – laceration, swelling. In my opinion, the report should have indicated an accidental fall outside, head hitting concrete, subsequent fall inside from dizziness, or something to that effect.

Now being transported to the hospital's emergency room for medical care, then followed by twenty-six days of non-remembered medical treatment, an emerging realization that I may not ever be the same person again came over me.

Hospital Bound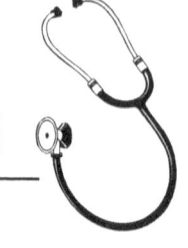

Once in emergency room care at a long-standing medical facility in the south end of West Palm Beach, an ER doctor took over with preliminary procedures. Later that day, a doctor of osteopathy (DO) was assigned as my attending physician. His position was as a hospitalist, one who handles clinical issues of patients, and most importantly, oversees their cases.

The attending physician was not board certified in any specialty at that time. He was tasked with overall responsibility for coordinating my care and treatment. I later found he had finished his medical education in what I would call a hodge-podge manner. He completed an associate of arts degree from Palm Beach Community College in 2004 and received state medical board licensing in 2012, with various educational venues in between.

To distinguish between doctors of osteopathy and medical doctors, sources say a DO focuses on whole body healing and has extra training in a technique known as osteopathic manipulated medicine. An MD generally focuses on treating specific conditions with medication. To note, in twenty-six days I had at least thirty-six different doctors, both DOs and MDs, performing their various care services. Fifteen of those doctors were consultants. I'm sorry, I don't remember any of you. My thoughts on this: Too many cooks, yada, yada and "Ka-ching."

The recorded diagnosis was quite unmelodramatic, in my opinion. Fall, syncope (pronounced syn-ka-pea), and leukocytosis. Fall is a vague diagnostic description. Did anyone in the ER ask what happened? At least Fire Rescue was a little more specific in their report, although somewhat lacking. Syncope means fainting with loss of consciousness. It may have been observed by Fire Rescue enroute to the hospital or by ER staff sometime after arriving; however, no specific qualifying entry was made of it in any record. Leukocytosis means a high white blood cell count as determined through a blood draw and testing. This could indicate a possible infection. Interestingly, research shows the condition may occur after a head injury.

Racking up almost nine hours in the emergency room following the morning's trauma, I must have been doubly distressed. I had scans, X-rays, IV insertions and lab work. A compression device for circulation and a heart monitor were ordered. I also had an additional electrocardiogram, the first being given in the rescue vehicle.

It may have been protocol to administer narcan, the anti-overdose drug, to incoming ER patients, just in case. However, by the time it was given to me more than three hours after arrival, I think overdosing would have been apparent. If it was a protocol, then rules are rules. Let it be shown record-wise that it was followed. I then had the drug's chaser, a medicine for possible side effects of nausea and vomiting. More than enough action for that long, first day. A room service meal was ordered at 9:41 p.m. There was no record of whether I ate anything.

Perhaps hunger triggered one of my false memories, quite a number of which I fabricated during my hospital stay. I was sitting at an old-fashioned school desk, seat attached to writing surface. A man facing a computer screen was sitting directly across from me. He had just finished my new patient processing. I told him I needed something to eat. "Pickin's will be scarce this time of day," he said. I noticed the spacious area we were in and didn't see much activity going on. He got up and went to see what he could find.

On returning, he placed a half sandwich, wrapped like those from a vending machine, on my school desktop. To go with it was a can of soda and a snack-size bag of the little fish-shaped cheese crackers. I was so grateful. Beyond parched, I immediately started chugging down the soda. Next came the sandwich. I took a bite. "Ugh!" One thin slice of turkey on dry wheat bread. No mayo. Nothing. Not worth eating. The crackers surprised me. How did he know I had recently acquired a taste for them, I wondered. The memory ended.

No Menu Needed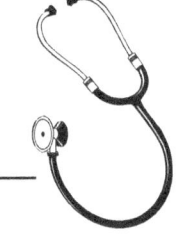

The syncope diagnosis became a stickler with medical staff on day one, then more so on day two, as I was having trouble swallowing. Could I have had a stroke-like event? That was where the focus seemed to be.

The attending physician had ordered a cardiology consult late on day one. It appeared the consultant was a no-show on day two. Maybe he phoned. There was no documentation of that. A second, on-staff doctor now stepped up to the plate. He seemed to be taking over the roles of both an attending physician and a primary care physician (PCP). I didn't have a PCP at the time. My usual doctor's office had left patients in the lurch while new people were taking over and getting clearance from insurance providers.

The second doctor will be referred to as my stand-in. He ordered repeat and additional tests, including an MRI. Putting first things first, I have a pacemaker implant, and an MRI scan lacked compatibility with a pacemaker at that time. I could have pointed that out. Surely, the record should have shown I had a pacemaker. Am I right? Using due diligence, the radiologist called the device manufacturer and canceled the order. I noticed the cancellation order had been placed in my record.

Unbelievably, over a week later another doctor ordered an MRI. Did he read my history, notes, anything at all? Apparently not. The doctor's name never again appeared in my records. In and out with a blink of an eye. A second MRI cancellation order was processed.

I was curious about how the CT (computer tomography) scan, which had already been done, differed from the MRI (magnetic resonance imaging). I learned the CT scan uses X-rays, whereas the

MRI uses electromagnetism, making it a no-no for me. My head CT showed no evidence for acute traumatic intracranial injury. The MRI is costlier, noisier, and said to show a bit more detail. Would the MRI have shed more light on my case? There is no way of knowing. Today, compatible MRI/pacemaker scan systems are available.

Muddying up the water now was the issue of non-swallowing. Termed dysphagia, the condition set an alarm off for new orders. A stroke coordinator was called, although no stroke had been confirmed. Swallowing therapy, plus a care plan, were put on the agenda. And a consultant would evaluate me for placing a tube into my stomach for feeding. Dysphagia is caused by damaged neurons (nerve cells) that control and coordinate throat muscles to allow swallowing. My research showed it is a common problem associated with traumatic brain injury. Two other causes are stroke and dementia.

This was another fine mess calling out for a mind manufactured memory. I was standing in a cubby-hole sized room, walls all white and completely bare, giving me no indication of my whereabouts. I was not in a hospital gown. A woman was facing me holding a teaspoon of what I assumed to be applesauce to my mouth. I was tasked with swallowing it. I couldn't. I spit out whatever she had spooned in. This internalized recollection was short and to the point.

After two days in the medical facility, it became clear I would not be an in-and-out patient, probably to the vexation of my healthcare insurance provider whose business model relies on keeping people out of hospitals.

With another order for a consultant and many more to come, I wanted to know about their function in the medical arena. The term itself conjures up reassurance. It raises expectations and trust. Resources say medical consultants are senior level, hospital-based physicians or surgeons who have completed their specialist training and are called in for surgery or difficult cases. Supposedly, the attending physician is to give the consultant a case summary, then communicate directly with the specialist to clarify notes and avoid misunderstanding. A written report should then be entered into the record giving a clear solution. In large part, what I first found were handwritten snippets tucked in here and there and test result findings written in medispeak. I later discovered that consultant reports had not been included in my request for ALL records, another snafu to deal with. In one instance a consultant had been called by phone and later contacted a nurse to fill him in as he was unfamiliar with the case.

Going forward, I had now become the "NPO" patient, meaning nothing by mouth from Latin nils per os. I started swallowing therapy given by speech therapists (ST) and continued with physical therapy (PT). This patient was not on an R&R track." I'm O.K.," a comment I made in ST, seemed to reassure everybody about my mental state after receiving the new diagnosis. Physical therapy notes stated "Muscle weakening with a good deal of assistance required for mobility tasks." It seemed there was no questioning of why I was losing motor and muscular functions. A mind boggler for me was that having had some incontinence while exercising, there was no hospital policy to clothe such patients in absorbent, hygienic underwear while in PT. Several of my sessions were canceled because "I had to be cleaned up." Patients do have pride.

"When had I stopped swallowing?" I wondered. As stated previously, a 9:41 p.m. meal was ordered on May 10. Did I eat? No record. Then at 11:42 p.m., two bedtime, by-mouth tablets were requested. As an NPO order was submitted at 12:46 a.m. on May 11, my guess is I could not swallow the pills. The hospital procedure, I believe, is to have a patient wrist-banded with the NPO status. At 9:46 a.m., May 11, the morning doctor ordered another by-mouth tablet. Maybe NPO should have been written on my forehead using indelible ink.

Surgery Sidelined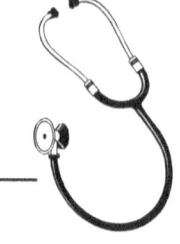

With a five-day empty belly, medical practice dictates getting nutrition into it, even if through a temporary nasogastric (NG) tube, or a permanently placed stomach tube called a PEG. The PEG procedure is lightweight in terms of risk. It involves using an endoscope, a tubular instrument inserted from the mouth to a hollow organ, mine being the stomach, to light it for viewing. The light could be seen from the stomach's exterior, thus pinpointing where to cut for tube insertion. Cut, place, it's over. I gave consent for a May 15 surgery. Unfortunately, the lead-in story to that event became way too complicated and resulted in a cancellation until May 17. The green signal for "go" quickly changed to red for "stop."

Before giving my version of the eventful days of May 15 and May 16, I feel compelled to express an opinion about my clinical records. They were as messy as an unkempt barnyard. I made a first attempt to learn how and by whom they were made without much success. Obviously, they were electronically generated, and again there appeared to be too many cooks making entries. A first example popped up right away. Notes were included about the correct positioning of a patient after having hip or knee replacement. It read like content for a teaching handbook and certainly didn't pertain to me. When and by whom the notes were entered will remain a mystery. A multitasker gone astray, perhaps? Additional and more serious missteps have been peppered throughout this tale. The quality of my care was beginning to look highly dubious.

Deciphering the chain of events leading to non-surgery exasperated me. I could have whittled my name twice on a walking stick in the time it took going over and over record entries. I began the day of May 15 with a blood pressure spike. My skin was pale, and my arms were described in terms more befitting a down-spiraling, 100-year-old woman. My arms had excess fluid. To note, an IV site had been leaking and was discontinued. Records showed that suspected/documented infection was answered yes, and antibiotic therapy was answered yes. Confusion over infection status reigned supreme throughout my hospitalization, with negatives sometimes contradicting positives and vice versa. Was a high white blood cell count reflecting brain injury or some other unnamed infection?

Leading to surgery, hourly oxygen was ordered. With this observation, "Bladder distended with discomfort," a Foley catheter was inserted. Brownish, maroon urine returned. A before surgery, operative assessment began. I stated the year was 2012 instead of 2017. Generalized musculoskeletal weakness was recorded, and the maroon urine was again referenced.

Shortly after 3:00 p.m., word was sent of surgery cancellation. High levels of two blood components that remove wastes from the kidneys were found indicating kidney failure. I found the following informative data from research which shows the complexity of my medical crisis. The kidney cleansing blood component, creatine, can be high after brain injury. A catheter can cause infection and blood in urine. Sepsis can lead to kidney failure. A puzzle, indeed. What was leading to what? This was the puzzle for physicians to solve.

Not to lose a minute, staff returned me to my usual hospital room to partake in PT and ST. Physical therapy noted "Fatigues easily." Speech (swallowing) therapy found a fungus called thrush in my mouth. In prior days, coughing and secretions had been building up, and now I had severe congestion. I asked for ice chips in ST, probably my only consolation. At some point, an infectious disease physician consult was ordered. The reason given: Elevated white blood cells and E. coli in urine.

So, another eventful day. Was it dinner time yet? Shortly before 8:00 p.m., a temporary nasogastric tube was placed for feeding.

Then came the bombshell medical record entry that five of my major body systems were marked yes for dysfunction resulting from severe sepsis. Those five were respiratory, cardiovascular, renal (kidney), metabolic, and hematologic systems. The hepatic (liver) and central nervous systems were marked no. My thought now about all the pathogens taking up residence in my body came from a humorous, but very applicable quote from the National Library of Medicine: "A dead host is a dead end." I was keeping all manner of them alive.

As a sidebar, the stand-in who involved himself in my case was called twice to report my surgery had been canceled. Records showed he never responded to those phone calls.

Cart Before the Horse

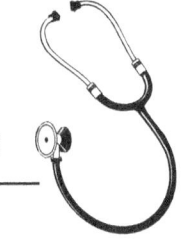

To break a moment from previously described hospital gloom, I'm putting the May 17 good news surgery cart first to overshadow the horse pulling it which had its own mercenary, pre-surgery agenda. The two-day fiasco ultimately resulted in a positive surgery outcome. The life-giving procedure to allow nutrients into my body was successfully performed and over by 9:10 a.m. on the seventeenth of May. Thanks go to the consultant/surgeon with the long, singsong Nigerian sounding name who did the deed. He left extensive record documentation behind as one would expect.

I learned, though, that feeding was not to start until the eighteenth. I had little to no nutrition for eight days, hardly a remedy for what ails you. Consulting with a retired nurse during medical-record examination, she questioned why the procedure hadn't been done sooner. My son-in-law, Dave, mentioned a doctor had told him non-swallowing would probably be temporary. The comment set off a blip of enlightenment within me. The doctor was still hanging on to the stroke diagnosis with its usual, short-lived dysphasia prognosis.

Dave again fit into my odyssey by appearing in another false memory. I was sitting in a hospital bed, railings up, with sheets scrunched all around me. I thought I was in my hospital's counterpart facility in the northern end of town. I must have heard "north" referenced at some point and incorporated that hospital in my mind. My family later nixed that remembrance. I was never there but had embodied it as a truth.

Continuing the memory, I was in an extremely spacious room with only one other bed so far to the left I was unsure if a patient was in it. All hospital staff were behind a concave glass enclosure doing whatever was required of them using computers and medical monitoring equipment. Dave was visiting me. He's a talker, sometimes repeating stories, but always engaging. He was telling me about his wristwatch – how it tracked his sleeping hours, how much time he spent in each stage of sleep, all manner of amazing data. He found it fascinating. Pointing to a white marker board with four names on it, he said three of the four named people would have tube placement surgeries that day. The fourth would be on the next day. The surgeon could only handle three a day, he told me.

I was the overnighter. It was a distressing one. I was freezing and couldn't get warm, no matter what I did. A loud racket kept coming from behind the wall on my right keeping me awake. Was it a hospital construction project? Alteration or renovation? I imagined what they might be doing. Carrying in lumber. Bringing in tools. But why at night? Just another false memory etched into my brain.

It's uncanny, but after many readings of the twenty plus records for the May 16, pre-surgery day, exact circumstances still elude me. My RN advisor was confused as well. Around 9:30 a.m., I was transferred from the intensive care unit to the respiratory unit. Shortness of breath and a chest X-ray indicated pulmonary congestion. A pulmonary consultant was called. A second thoracentesis order went in, the first sent earlier but not yet acted upon. Lab requests were made for examining the drawn fluid from my left lung. I was receiving oxygen via nasal cannula while in the respiratory unit.

At 11:02 a.m., Rapid Response was called. Here's when clinical records halted for an hour. What little I learned came from a very illegible, hand-written response team report and its short, typewritten counterpart. The team report was misdated, but its counterpart was correct. Boxes checked off showed I was not responding to treatment and was suctioned. What treatment was I having? Seeking clarification from the discharge report, it seemed I was having an aerosol treatment. I found no documentation of how it was being administered. The decipherable handwriting on the team report said I was worsening, wheezing, and had pulled out the (?) tube. The (?) tube was a two-letter abbreviation which I couldn't make out. The typewritten report said the team was called because of a lot of upper airway secretions. When they arrived, I was lethargic with what they noted as gurgling and crackles, but I was stable and suctioned.

At noon the thoracentesis procedure was done at bedside with about a cup of serous fluid being removed from my left lung. It was completed in less than one-half hour. Medical accounts went astray when describing supposed events related to tube pulling. In my case, unclear and insufficient documentation of tubes going in and tubes going out led to confusion. Scheduled ST therapy staff had received a cancellation note stating "Patient is not seen by ST secondary to PT (patient) Rapid Response." The note's comment read "Found with aspiration pneumonia. Patient pulled NG (nasogastric) tube and not appropriate for PEG placement." There was no record of the note sender. Winding down from the thoracentesis, records stated the "trumpet" was successfully removed. My RN advisor described the trumpet saying it was used to keep the airway open. I talked to her at length for clarification about the various tube insertions. She was confused as well and agreed there were many gaps in this part of record documentation. My analysis: I was not having an NG tube feeding while in the respiratory unit and therefore did not pull out the tube resulting in aspiration pneumonia. The staff's subjective, hand-to-hand comments do not suffice as properly documented medical records. Neither does an unaccounted for gap in clinical records, especially when a serious medical situation is happening.

Moving on, while lying on my side for the thoracentesis and wearing the back-opening hospital gown, pressure ulcers were noted on my buttocks. Wound consultation along with alleviating ulcer procedures were ordered. I will further expand on hospital buttock happenings in a later chapter. Nutrition management was next on the agenda. They were on target with a risk assessment that said "high," but had also received the comment of NG tube pulling. That comment did have labeling saying it was subjective. Again, my hospital day was endless. Now it was on to respiratory therapy. Their report stated my condition as being cardiopulmonary disease. Fifteen minutes of PT followed. Not a moment to lose!

My daughter Laura was with me in the hospital on both the sixteenth and seventeenth, having driven to West Palm Beach from Bonita Springs on Florida's west coast. I was not at all surprised when she quoted me to the nurse on the sixteenth as saying "I wanted to go home." Records showed that on the night of the seventeenth I was lethargic and mildly confused. And my daughter reported that I was attempting to climb out of bed.

Sepsis Overload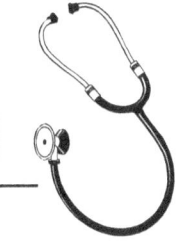

One day several years ago, I was surfing TV channels and stopped when hearing Whoopi Goldberg speaking in a pontifical-like manner about her experience with sepsis while appearing on a talk show. She warned of the severity of her sepsis response to infection while being treated for pneumonia. Her hospital in-patient stay could have been a typical four to five days for pneumonia. Instead, it was around a month, I believe, due to the often-fatal, sepsis toxicity. I had heard the word sepsis used in tandem with the phrase blood poisoning, an incorrect description according to the Sepsis Alliance. I paid no attention, as I had never known anyone who had it. Then Whoopi enlightened me.

On hospital day one in the ER, I had a sepsis screen, and a care coordinator was notified for good measure in case of a positive outcome. Establishing a patient as positive upon hospital entry would be beneficial for treatment and might negate suspicion of a hospital acquired infection resulting in sepsis. Record entries on my first day showed I had been started on two antibiotics given through an IV, which were not prophylactics. In other words, they were not preventative drugs to mitigate a bacterial infection that could be looming. This would suggest that I already had a medically verifiable infection upon hospital entry, which had not been established.

When I first read the word sepsis, I went ballistically overboard. Quickly, I grabbed a highlighter and began marking each page where the word appeared. The Sepsis Alliance states the condition as "The body's overwhelming and life-threatening response to infection that can lead to tissue damage, organ failure, and death." It kills around 350,000 Americans each year and 11 million worldwide.

Three days after the initial sepsis screen was made, record entries showed I was not positive for severe sepsis, and what is termed a sepsis bundle was not implemented. A bundle is a series of medical responses a physician team takes for treatment, including specific testing, IV fluids, and antibiotics. I have no idea how the bundle differed from the antibiotic treatment already in place. Forty-five minutes into the next shift the nurse again reported the circumstantial suspected/documented infection as yes, and antibiotic therapy as yes. Nowhere at this time did I find concrete, documented specifics about the source of this suspected infection. Uncertain record interpretation resulted from not knowing exactly what was yes, and what was no.

A day later, May 14, there was again no record of sepsis. Then the May 15 bombshell was dropped: renal failure, no scheduled PEG surgery for the insertion of a feeding tube, and five major body systems impaired by severe sepsis. I may have been trying to outrun the infection, but to no avail.

The Alliance states that severe sepsis survivors have an increased risk of a repeat episode. Records indicated sepsis was lingering during my hospital stay without being resolved. The morning of May 26 showed the following:

- Patient positive for severe sepsis/document bundle: Y.
- Date physician notified of positive sepsis screen: 05/26/17.
- Sepsis bundles implemented: No.
- If sepsis bundle not implemented, select primary reason: MD decision.

Then on June 2, four days before my discharge to a nursing home, I found this:

- Patient positive for severe sepsis/document bundle, yes.
- Nurses note, yes.

- Date physician notified of positive sepsis screen, 06/02/17.
- Sepsis bundles implemented, no.
- If sepsis bundle not implemented, select primary reason: MD decision.
- Severe sepsis comment: MD aware of condition.

I can only assume it was the stand-in making the decisions. Records do lack clarity.

After the last positive screening for sepsis, I was pushed out to a nursing home to either sink or swim. Knowing now the complete story of my hospital stay, I believe the transition to a nursing home may have been my saving grace, giving me a rest from the everything-under-the-sink medical bombardments thrown at me in the name of good medicine.

The Life After Sepsis Fact Sheet published by the Sepsis Alliance states "Up to 50% of sepsis survivors are left with physical and/or psychological long-term effects." Listed are many conditions that fall within the post-sepsis syndrome, some of which are insomnia, nightmares, and extreme fatigue. I can attest to having them all.

What became so excruciatingly painful to me, more so than the overall healthcare odyssey, was that neither of my two daughters were told about my serious sepsis condition. I asked them each three times. Nothing was said about it or its ramifications such as a high, ongoing mortality rate, or significantly lower quality of life for survivors. I had asked Anne about conversations we had during visiting hours. She said, "You were pretty much out of it," thinking it may have been from medications. In fact, with sepsis you may become confused, sleepy, and difficult to rouse according to the Alliance.

I found out the medical facility was a teaching hospital, at least at that time. Perhaps that's why so many doctors were prancing around me, willy-nilly, hoping to enhance their own career by solving unknown medical mysteries. What I needed was a team of first-rate, highly experienced physicians at bedside specifically focused on my own illness.

There is one thing I can wholly agree with as stated by a nurse in James Patterson's book, *E.R. Nurses.* "Hospitals are dirty places."

Apologies All 'round

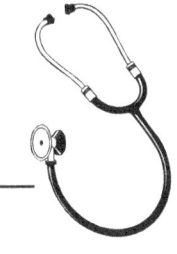

R ecord retrieval from storage became another sticking point when writing *Brainwreck*. In my first request for records, I asked for everything – everything as in all, the whole and complete quantity, or "kit and caboodle," so to speak. What's not to understand? When I received my yardstick-high box, I assumed the request had been fulfilled. No so. Imagine my astonishment when later requesting several clinical record duplicates, I instead found never yet seen consultant reports. How was I to deal with this? I had already written seven chapters. I may owe an apology, then, to consultants whom I might have offended by off-the-cuff remarks made in previous chapters.

However, preliminary record examination of this new information suggested my remarks had been substantially sound. What I discovered was more than enough documentation to support my insight into hospital decision making. Sometimes medical calls were on the mark. At other times they were so outrageous they could have been labeled as incompetent. Histories, Impressions, and Findings were ping-ponged about among hospital generalists and specialists, each putting their own tweak or spin on the medicinal ball as my case evolved. Opinions ebbed and flowed through way too many medical professionals unfamiliar with my circumstances going back to day one.

One intriguing example made by a doctor and entered into the automated clinical record referenced parkinsonism. A family member has the neurological disorder Parkinson's, so I was familiar with its dynamics. However, I had to consult my medical dictionary for clarification of the word parkinsonism. Indeed, parkinsonism can result from brain injury. I recalled, though, its manifestation was relative to repeated head trauma, usually sustained in sports. The comment ping-ponged later when two consultants stated I had Parkinson's, or alternatively parkinsonism, which I did not have.

To deal with the inclusion of new material, I've had to mesh it with already written material to more accurately reflect circumstances from hospital day one to after PEG surgery. The remaining, newly provided material will mesh with the narrative as it proceeds. Record request confusion could be a fitting metaphor for my entire, twenty-six-day hospitalization.

On day one in the emergency room, I complained of pain in the areas impacted by the fall only, with no other discomforts except weakness. I stated I was confused and dizzy, which abated in around two hours. Head and pelvic CTs showed no abnormalities, except for a tiny "bone island" found on the pelvis. This finding turned into another ping-pong quest as will be described in a later chapter. X-rays of the chest and elbow showed no abnormalities.

The mysterious suspected/documented infection described earlier came from the day-one ER report stating I was given antibiotics for an unknown infection, subjectively labeled urinary tract infection, although I reported no symptoms.

The head laceration was not recognized as anything consequential. After two hours in the ER, the wound was tended to with five staples, five stitches, and copious irrigation. With an estimated length of four inches, it was described as large in one report and termed small in a consultant report. Swelling went unnoted until the next day; however, the emergency response team had documented the area as swollen when I was being transported to the hospital.

With an abnormal EKG, diagnoses of stroke, syncope, ischemia, and TIA, all heart related conditions, were bandied about. I denied syncope as well as chest pain. Picking up on and carrying through all records was that term, syncope, which was leading team players to the wrong ballpark. Surely, the word stroke under the caption

History on my second brain CT exam report did that as well. I had not had a stroke. But hey, let's give her a stress test. Test summary, "The stress EKG was negative for ischemia and normal." Here's when I first realized it would be highly beneficial to standardize and correlate consultant records with exam report records.

On May 15, severe sepsis bombshell day, a consultant was called to evaluate me for the ongoing high white cell blood count. The consultant's report stated I was not a good informer; I was confused. That seemed likely with a severe sepsis diagnosis. Her lengthy writeup came mostly from chart review, she noted. Under the caption Impression, she stated a deep abscess infection could be considered although "Findings on the exam would be surprising for that." She recommended I continue with the antibiotic currently being given. Beware of the word abscess, another ping-pong in the making.

I was not able to decipher the time or circumstances of the consultant's visit and why no mention of sepsis was made in her report. It had been documented in the clinical record that same day. She did make a remark about my irregular, irregular heartbeat. That fact was true and probably still is. At this stage of my life, I do not fear it and will not seek treatment. My choice.

A second apology is now due to *me* from the hospital's record storage providers. Changes made with record providers ultimately resulted in contracting with a large, out-of-state company. Coalescing methods between the two providers seemed not to be in sync. You'll not be surprised to learn that after a second request for the same document duplicates, I again received something never seen before. Issues with receiving records speak poorly of medical record providers.

Decisions, Decisions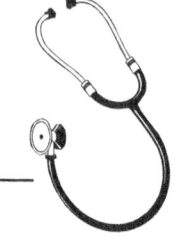

Now with a means of feeding in place, thought was given to my readiness for hospital discharge. The stand-in doctor ordered a case management consultation for discharge planning. He, too, was hodge-podge educated and in my opinion had made inaccuracies of fact, reasoning, and judgment. I am not suggesting the call was inappropriate, as at this step it may have been procedural. However, it did not stop him from continuing to batter me with additional testing, applicable or not, and all a part of the leave no stone unturned mentality.

My understanding of a discharge plan is that hospital staff and insurance providers coordinate to determine a patient's readiness to leave the hospital, then follow through with getting the individual on to the next step. That may be a skilled nursing facility or home care with caretakers in place. Decision making can be a slippery slope. It may free up a needed hospital bed on the one hand, or on the other may risk a patient's return to expensive hospital care if not medically ready.

Along with discharge planning came something called neurological deconditioning. A consultant was called to perform this readiness procedure. With the aid of a medical dictionary and other sources, my interpretation was that because I had eight hospital days under abnormal physiological conditions from illness and immobility, I would need to be reprogrammed. The goal would be to have me normally receive and interpret stimuli that transmit impulses to responsive organs. I found no record of these orders taking place or being canceled. In hindsight, deconditioning would have been a folly under my sepsis and undiagnosed brain injury circumstances. How could my body have been responsive in any way, shape, or form?

Not to miss a beat, thyroid testing was next on the agenda. I doubted whether a malfunctioning thyroid could have contributed to any aspect of my illness. But I suppose finding a glitch would be a doctor win. No glitch was found. However, my potassium level needed a boost, so all was not lost. This was the day the in-and-out doctor from nowhere ordered the second MRI which was canceled.

Quagmired in discordant rhyme or reason, an additional order subjected me to another questionable undertaking. A whole-body bone scan was ordered. Had they mixed me up with another patient? It happens. Under exam History the report stated, "Fall, cancer, unspecified metastases." Unbelievable. I had no cancer, therefore could have no metastases. Is my thinking incorrect? Where had this off-base history come from? It took me awhile to figure out the mess. Going back to hospital day one, a CT was made of my cervical spine to rule out fracture. That scan report stated a tiny density was found in the spine (spine area named), possibly a bone island, as I mentioned previously. Also noted was that further consideration of a follow-up be made if there was concern about the possibility of osteoblastic metastatic disease. Of course, I also had to look up this terminology.

Osteoblastic metastases develop when cancer cells invade the bone and cause too many bone cells to form. Again, I had no primary cancer for cells to break away from. A bone island is a tiny piece of bone that lodges in another section of bone and is noncancerous. No matter. We're off to another raucous "Ka-ching" event, a nuclear medicine scan. It uses a radioactive substance called a tracer, which after being intravenously injected, highlights areas where it is absorbed and appears on the scan. It was not a short procedure. The scan showed nothing of consequence. Then, another stone turning was recommended, "Correlation with pelvic CT with IV contrast," meaning an additional nuclear medicine scan.

Why am I not surprised that the new recommendation took a curiously odd turn. The next day an abdominal/pelvis CT with contrast was ordered. Exam History stated abdominal pain, unspecified abdominal mass. My reaction when reading this – Huh! What happened to the follow up to osteoblastic metastatic disease. I believe the pendulum had swung back to the infectious disease consultant's report of May 15 mentioning an unlikely, deep abscess infection. So here we go with an alternative nuclear medicine scan. Just another ping-pong event. The Exam Impression stated "No acute abdominopelvic inflammatory process identified."

Another little addition to the constant injection needle pokes, IV's, and blood draws came with an injection that inhibits gastric acid secretion. It had been given in response to the passage of a dark stool. Perhaps a result of PEG surgery two days earlier and start of feeding tube use one day after? Perhaps something to monitor? Or maybe just overkill? The medication had strict criteria for use, none of which applied. Filled in for Other Indication was melena, or dark stool indicating decomposing blood. The beat goes on.

Hospital Continuum

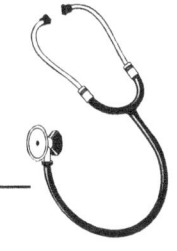

With hospital staff agreeing with one thing only, that I was still critically ill and very weak, discharge was off the table. Eleven days had passed, and now it was time for two more consultations – one a psychiatrist consult for depression, the other a pulmonologist for shortness of breath and lung fluid. Both doctors saw me on the same day.

The psychiatrist's consultation report reflected my comment made to him that my antidepressant was "Working pretty well," which was noted under chief complaint. In other words, I didn't have a complaint. So why was the consultant called? Then, the ubiquitous medical term, parkinsonism, crept into his report as mentioned earlier. Here's where my sense of being in good hands became further eroded. His report stated that "An alternative drug for depression (medication named) may be a better match for her parkinsonism." Then he noted he would leave medications as they were.

The second consultant for lung issues floored me. Not since reading the word sepsis early on in my clinical records had I felt so beleaguered by seemingly substandard medical practice. His report, under a listing of Other History said, "She also has Parkinson's." He wrote a list of six recommendations. Number five stated the following: "Would hold off on scopolamine in light of neurologic diagnosis." Scopolamine? I had to scour through medical resources to find a meaning or description of the term. Finally, I found one that would suit his affirmation of Parkinson's: Used as an agent that affects nerve transmission. And what about a neurologic diagnosis? Was he prompting one, or just looking back at the order for one eight days into hospitalization that never happened? The one for neurological deconditioning for discharge?

How did this derailment take place? I can only assume the specialists had not been given an adequate case summary. Nor had they communicated with the attending physician or his stand-in who called most of the shots. Or maybe the two consultants were consulting with each other making two wrongs a right. In any case, I will now defiantly proclaim I did not have Parkinson's then; I do not have it now. Quickly we moved on, leaving another fiasco behind.

The next day the portable, upright chest radiograph came calling, along with its attendant, to take another chest X-ray. The X-ray showed views like the one taken after my thoracentesis six days earlier. Having discussed the contents of the exam report with my RN advisor, mild pneumonia was the culprit.

Another chest X-ray two days later, with little change and white blood cell count remaining high, the pulmonary doctor spoke to my daughter of his concern. He was hesitant to try a stronger medication, then acquiesced. He started me on the empiric drug mentioned earlier – a seven-day regime of injections. I expect with some awareness of non-response chitchat by medical staff, my mind fabricated another memory to soothe the soul. It seemed real enough. However, when I later asked my daughter about it, she said it didn't happen.

I recall I was in a wheelchair. Anne was behind me with the doctor beside us. We were grouped with others, all looking up at a huge screen mounted on the wall. Patient's names and statistics were slowly scrolling downward giving viewers time to read them. The doctor was waiting for mine to appear. When he saw it, he was pleased, indicating to Anne that the white blood cell count had lowered. It had lowered in my false memory only.

Somewhere during the time frame of the pneumonia debacle, the stitches and staples from my mostly unnoticed, unmeaningful, and inaccurately corroborated head wound were removed.

Now on the May 26 agenda, a hematologist (blood doctor) was

to be summoned to evaluate leukocytosis management. On the minus side, the erroneous "Frequent falls at home" statement was reiterated in the physician's report. On the plus side, Parkinson's and parkinsonism had become moot points. I reported to him that I was "not great" and had not been out of bed. With his review of that day's chest and abdominal/pelvic exams, he indicated infectious disease was unlikely.

The Molecular Genetics JAK2 V617F Mutation Analysis was another rock to turn, so it was ordered. I cannot imagine how the referral reason; syncope, fall, could have even substantiated such a costly, chromosomal test. By now, though, it seemed not to matter what referrals, histories, or other criteria were stated for exam requests. Maybe the only need was to have an MD or DO behind one's name. On behalf of the hematologist, he ultimately did state in his report that the test was to rule out a leukemic disorder, or words to that effect.

With a big "Ka-ching" resounding, no mutation was detected.

Urointrigues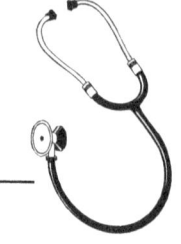

Looking back at doctor suggested or perceived maladies, plus the correctly diagnosed ones, I concluded many came to an impasse before resolution. One suspected malady would pop up to supersede a prior one before any conclusion was recorded. The focus kept changing with no end in sight. Who was on the diagnostic treadmill? Everyone, it seemed, including the exhausted patient. The next phase of hospitalization involved all things urologic. Liquid in, liquid out. Seemed so simple. It always had been. Now it was becoming a problem. It rolled right into another memory fabrication.

I was attending a health fair which was set up in a sparsely grassed field. Instead of tables or booths, brown army tents were haphazardly erected, and visitors could enter to pick up brochures and speak with representatives. I entered one tent and was directed to another. I was told I needed a urinalysis. Once in the next, somewhat hard to find tent, someone spoke to me saying in no uncertain terms, "You cannot have a urinalysis." The reason given was because I had urinary retention. I didn't know what to do and stood there puzzled and in a dither. The actual hospital events of May 27, 28, and beyond played out this memory.

Before entering the urophase, I find it relevant to mention more of the previous day's affairs. The clinical report again noted I was positive for sepsis. A sepsis bundle had not been implemented per MD decision, which I assumed was by my stand-in. Records showed I was confused, forgetful, and disoriented to time. My breathing was labored. That was the day of the hematologist's visit. His report stated "There is no evidence of an ID process on cultures of blood, urine, and pleural fluid in this hospitalization." If the comment was accurate, I wondered how it might have had a bearing on my case or if an ID process was considered standard practice. Further, he stated "From his perspective she may be released to rehabilitation."

A new malady quickly came on from my complaint of abdominal pain; however, I could not find at what time I had reported it. Starting very early on May 27, medical prancing on my behalf began. At 1:45 a.m., an on-staff doctor for the day ordered a chest CT scan. Was it a follow-up for pneumonia? Why was it ordered so early? Another doctor put a hold on PEG tube feeding at 7:42 a.m. Perhaps because of the abdominal pain report? While in respiratory therapy at 9:48 a.m., another doctor ordered the use of a small device to remove mucous while I was having nebulizer treatments.

The same 1:45 a.m. doctor, now informed of the abdominal pain report, added an abdominal/pelvic scan with contrast, to the roster of orders. At about that time, 11:00 a.m., my stand-in came aboard and requested that lab work be done. The attending physician had always kept me supplied with oxygen canisters, one of his few contributions, but on that day another doctor ordered it. Perhaps the supply was diminishing faster than calculated. With all the names of this doctor and that doctor, I surmised it must have been a special, pinch-hitter weekend. It certainly was – Memorial Day weekend, 2017.

By late afternoon, the whirlwind atmosphere had not calmed. Readying me for scan procedures, another pinch hitter ordered the contrast agents to be used for the scans. One would be administered by IV, the other through the PEG tube going directly into my stomach. Off I went to partake in the magic power of scanning science.

Scan news was not good news. It showed a left pelvic area fluid collection of notable size. Plus, there was "New marked urinary bladder distention." I learned through my research that sepsis can cause bladder distention. My stand-in ordered catheter placement, followed by a surgical physician consult, naming a specific doctor. The reason: Perforated viscus. This could be a serious situation, depending on circumstances. There was a no connect with that doctor, again a holiday weekend. So that order was canceled.

Efforts continued to find another consultant, this time from urology. Ordering snafus such as wrong doctor or no signature held up progress. Two telling outcomes came from that day's events involving around nine doctors, including the pinch hitters. Blood testing ordered by the stand-in revealed more fungi feasting – perhaps a holiday bar-b-que? An IV bag of antifungal medication was started. Then the kicker. Over a two-hour period, 2,000 ml, or 67 ounces, or 8 cups of urine, were drained by catheter from my bladder. Typically, a female bladder holds two cups during the day and four at night. I will leave you to ponder about the fluid collection shown in the pelvic scan and how it got there. In my view, something had to give.

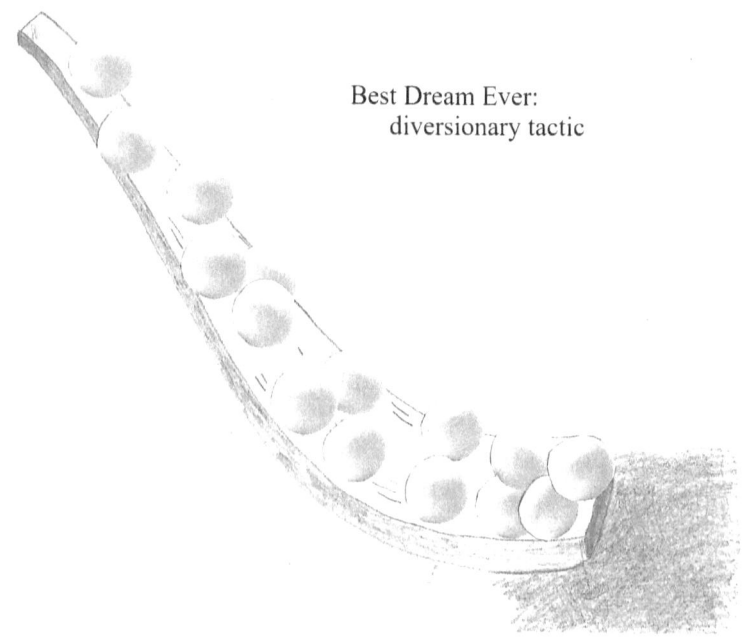

Best Dream Ever:
diversionary tactic

Standoffs

Record-wise, urology events were a bit sketchy. Noted in the clinical record on May 27, an in-house doctor spoke with me about surgery for pelvic fluid removal. I refused to have it. By this time who knows what my mind was latching onto.

By May 28, a urology consultant had come on board. He had discussed my case with another physician who told him the fluid was amenable to percutaneous (cutting through skin) drainage. The consultant posed the procedure to me as being an intervention. By now, my body/mind connection must have felt overdosed with medical mania. I told the doctor, "I had too many interventions and would not take anymore." As I no longer had pain or abdominal tenderness, I must have wanted to be left alone.

The doctor went on to ask if I understood the implications. I nodded yes. To clarify he asked, "Are you ready to go to heaven?" I nodded yes. This prompted a most profound dream capturing the standoff dilemma. I was a flannel ball, a little smaller than a soccer ball. The flannel was soft, like a newborn baby's hospital blanket, but without pink and blue striping. I was among many other white flannel balls on a slightly sloped conveyer chute which fed into a dark opening. They would soon be coming to find me, I knew. I kept repositioning myself further down on the chute making myself harder to find. For now, I was safe. But I knew they would soon find me.

Now my stand-in was ready for his own standoff. Or was it his stand-down? It came in the form of a discharge summary written on May 29. Discharge summaries, I learned, are written by junior doctors, usually using templates. A hospital may have its own template to simplify procedures. This summary exemplified to me there was no grasp of the extent, causes, and ramifications of my hospitalization, and I doubt if the summary would have been meaningful to anyone. Errors were repeated such as stroke, and spelling was atrocious. Still, it was a bona-fide record and had an addendum attached to it by yet another doctor.

The next two days seemed to be ones of lying low, with no major upending by another malady. Still, sepsis remained. Probably the down time, except for therapies, was a balm to the brain, as brain injured people need significantly more rest and significantly less activity.

On the morning of May 31, I was still refusing the proposed intervention, but later relented and gave consent. Again, leukocytosis lent itself to describing the procedure as the drainage of an abscess, or a pocket of infection. This had been an assumption. Of course we were traversing through doctors without a guidepost.

The pelvic drainage report noted I tolerated the procedure well. It was uneventful, and I was stable. But I was perplexed by the data giving the accounting of time for the surgery. One accounting said I was administered conscious sedation and a tranquilizer at 4:34 p.m. Both were given again at around 5:15 p.m. Late doctor? I had to try to correlate that with the exam report's start time of 17:35 (5:35 p.m.) and going backwards to the end time of 16:15 (4:15 p.m.). Total time, 18 minutes. No amount of higher math is going to help me out with this one.

The days after the circuitous urointrigues were dedicated to hospital discharge. It had been scheduled for June 6. Follow-up scans and various medigrams were put on the agenda. One scan was for pneumonia, now termed respiratory failure, the other for bladder rupture, now acknowledged as such. Another pesky X-ray, a cystogram, was taken to rule out an abnormality of the bladder. No stone unturned. Tabs on my creatine levels had been kept, this relative to proper kidney functioning.

The stand-in physician had basically bowed out since writing the discharge summary on May 29. A few other doctors took over, part and parcel, to see me out the door. The few who may have been following my case might have concluded that I had been overrun by sepsis, I was antibiotic resistant, and my future was uncertain. All true, but with a big missing piece. My brain had also been traumatized by a fall.

Abomination or Absolution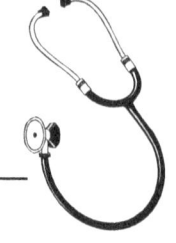

M edical record examination slowly evolved into my own intellectual sport, although an extremely tiring one. Traversing through myriad data with dots unconnected, mazes obscured, and questionable reasoning, I was forced to make sense of it all to achieve my goal.

I'm not medically schooled and believe I have had less interaction with medical professionals than others my age, until the time of my fall. But my analytical ability remained highly intact. It gave me an edge in deciphering the nature of my complex illness and the missteps it engendered.

I was amazed by the number of assessments, goals to reach, and standards of care to be met that bulked up the clinical records. All mandated by prestigious hospital and state boards to assure best practices for patients, I expect. But implementing evaluative measures is only as good as the observational and reasoning skills of the medical staff using them and the educational and experiential background of those who create them. I had way too many evaluative record entries to muse over.

One process was named the Braden Pressure Ulcer Risk Assessment, which seemed to have forsaken me in determining my risk. I had seen a photographic wound sheet floating around in my records. An anatomical sketch of the body's backside was shown with the buttocks circled. Mine? Then I found a consecutive, four-day ulcer risk rating while waiting for the PEG tube placement and having no feedings: May 13 – high risk, nutrition poor; May 14 – mild risk, nutrition adequate; May 15 (sepsis doomsday) – low risk, adequate nutrition; May 16 – high risk, very poor nutrition. Does this make sense? It didn't to me.

I had another quibble with the ulcer wound sheet. It was missing information. The signature, date, and time were illegible, except for the name Maria, and how many Marias are out there. The sheet was date-stamped by the attending physician on June 24, 2017, eighteen days after my discharge to a nursing home. Excellent memory or just a misdated authentication stamp?

The policy for not using absorbent hygiene products for incontinence, occasional or otherwise, also stymied me. I called the hospital for their take on the matter. The answer was they felt the use of diapers, or nappies (as I prefer to call them), on mostly bedridden patients contributed to pressure ulcer development. It didn't seem to work for me. I say choose nappies over the unhygienic soiling and cleaning up afterward alternative. Call bells are slow to be answered.

Therapy staff also entered copious notes, assessments, and recommendations. They were adequately descriptive and comprehensive. I had finally learned some ins and outs of record generation from my RN advisor. Electronic screens are accessed to allow for filling in of the particulars as matched to the record type, such as clinical or physical therapy, etc. A generic response can be made from a list, or comments specific to the case can be inserted. In two cases, I noted a therapist had recommended a diagnostic avenue for the doctor to explore. My RN advisor said this was professionally acceptable and, in fact, could be helpful.

There were so many patient status record entries it led me to wonder whether nurses had time to review and question prior ones. Ongoing related medical connections might have been recognized with more time to do so. And with so much to review, were they able to focus on the present day's overview. Documented entries included vitals, skin, vascular, neurological, gastrointestinal, and so on. At some point in the record, nurses and therapists had to give an attestation affirming they had followed certain Standards of Care, something that is mandated, I presume. Are they going to say no?

When I pictured my overall hospital experience years later, I formed the image of a train derailment as seen from overhead. A panoramic sky view of overturned railcars, off-track and zigzaggedly askew seemed the best visual likeness. Only through my own long and laborious research was this comparison made apparent. When leaving the hospital, there was uncertainty whether I would ever again be in good health. The odds were not in my favor, and only time would tell.

My traumatic brain injury (TBI) remained professionally undiagnosed for over three years. TBI is sometimes referred to as a silent injury and is the least understood cause of death in the United States. It was only when I was well enough to see a recommended neurologist that the diagnosis was confirmed. All I had to say was that I was hospitalized for twenty-six days after a head injury and didn't remember any of it. I added that the only thing I had for memories were a good number of false ones.

Surely, hospital doctors should have had an inkling of the relational aspect of head injury to dysphasia and ambulatory disfunction. Brain messaging had been disrupted. That had become my opinionated stance. No one mentioned the possibility of brain injury to my daughters. If someone on staff had, I know they would have sought out appropriate sources for a better understanding of my condition and behavior. I remember saying to my daughter when she was visiting me in assisting living, "Something is wrong with me, and somebody better find out." I had also said to her at one time, "I feel like a freak."

The thrust of my long illness came from severe sepsis. I can only describe it as evil, in the harshest sense of the word. If you don't die from it, you may well wish you had. Specific information about its manifestation was hard to find. At best, it can be described as a response to infection wherein the immune system releases toxic chemicals into the bloodstream. This causes inflammation throughout the body, possibly resulting in organ dysfunction or failure. The Sepsis

Alliance states sepsis is the leading cause of death in United States' hospitals. The Alliance is an advocate for developing newer, effective antibiotics for treatment and reducing overuse of the existing ones.

There is no certainty about how and when I acquired sepsis. The National Institute of Health says patients with traumatic brain injury are susceptible to sepsis which may exacerbate the systemic inflammatory response. Alternatively, it may have resulted from a healthcare-acquired infection from one of the many invasive devices used in treatment such as IVs, urinary catheters, injection devices, and tubes. It is unfathomable how severe sepsis was medically verified yet remained virtually unspoken of among the medical staff caretaking me.

I have formed my own diagnosis of why I became critically ill, and that was my goal. I'm satisfied with my conclusion. Three major culprits were to blame: TBI, severe sepsis, and the ongoing, relentless bombardment of the hospital's leave-no-stone-unturned methodology. Can there be too much medicine? Yes, too many doctors and doctor orders, too many drugs, too many opinions and exams, too many injections, IVs, and therapies.

Could I have had liquid Robitussin with codeine as prescribed by one in-and-out doctor? No, I was NPO. Could I have had an MRI? No, but it was twice ordered by separate doctors. Did I have Parkinson's? Definitely not. This was the real derailment – medical disconnection.

In September 2023, six years after my hospitalization, my mind put to rest any remaining anguish that I felt since my trauma. In a frightening nightmare, an indistinct ghoulish monster was approaching me, coming from nowhere. Closer and closer it came. To do me harm. I tried to scream, again and again. Nothing came out of my mouth. Closer and closer it came. Finally, at the end of the dream the scream began to erupt. I popped awake and sat up in terror. I expected to be screaming. It took me awhile to process the occurrence. Then I knew. It was a final purging.

II

NURSING HOME

New Lodgings

I t was the proverbial dark and stormy night when I was discharged
to a skilled nursing facility, commonly called a nursing home. The
sky had opened its floodgates sending pelting sheets of rain, with
accompanying loud, thunderous bolts of lightning. South Florida's
subtropical summer weather was in full swing. The move to a new
care home was not a seamless one.

My daughter Anne was in the hospital with me while I was
being readied for transport. This I do recall, as my memory
was beginning to return. The nurse decided or was instructed
to start a feeding before transit by ambulance as schedules and
paperwork snafus could hold up the best of plans. The nurse was
having trouble with the connector tube and pouch of milk, as
the liquid was sometimes called. She must have had a long day
as she became frustrated with trying to get everything to work.
She then threw the feeding paraphernalia into the transport bed
I was in and left.

The ambulance came and off my daughter and I went. The trip
was long and slow with the storm raging and work to home traffic
clogging the roadway. My daughter was encouraging me and helping
to keep me calm as we juggernauted from lane to lane as impatient
drivers will often do.

Once inside the facility, my memory again became skewed with
another half-true recollection. I was at the entry area, still in the hospital bed, with my dinner accoutrements bedded with me. Several
staffers in uniforms were gathered around me. Looking down at me,
they were whispering back and forth. Then I heard one softly say,
"We can't take her here." My daughter later told me there had been

an issue with the feeding tube. It had been clogged. A night shift nurse was soon rounded up who sorted it all out.

Morning came. I had not been booted out. This led to my last fabricated recollection. Dressed in a nightgown, I was standing on my own looking around my new home. Flowered wallpaper borders just below the ceiling enhanced the room. So typically facility-like. It was a Sunday. I heard hymnal singing nearby. There must be a small auditorium just down the hall with steps leading up to a double-doored entrance. I could picture it. Welcoming. Nice place for activities – bingo and such. However, I could not stand, walk, or much less play bingo, so I questioned what my days might be like.

Thinking back to that first nursing home day and now into the research phase of my odyssey, I was curious to know what information had been passed on to the facility about my care needs. Record requests can run afoul with long wait times, so I asked the facility for them early on in my writing project. Yes, the request did go afoul in more ways than one. Over two months later, I received word that the nursing home had changed hands and past patient records were no longer there. I had to assume, then, that the hospital discharge records supplied to me were identical to those supplied to them.

From the discharge instructions, the original hospital admittance diagnosis of fall, syncope, and leukocytosis remained. Nothing else. Why would this lead to nursing home care? The instruction sheet said I could resume previous activity. Well, I did. Critically ill and in a hospital bed. Under surgery procedures I had while hospitalized, stomach tube placement surgery was listed twice. Apparently, the actual procedure plus the canceled one were both listed. I wonder if my health insurance paid twice or picked up on the mistake avoiding a double whammy.

Two other invasive procedures were not noted. On page 171 of the 174-discharge report, it again stated I could resume previous activity as well as return to work/school. Under the question "Does patient have any of the following conditions," the answer was none.

There was no list of conditions on the record sheet, but they could be viewed on a hospital screen. So sure thing, I could return to work/school. Covid was not yet in the picture.

My daughter had received copies of prescriptions to hand over to the facility. Her comment "You aren't on many drugs," surprised me. It seemed that most of my medications were given intravenously due to my NPO status. If given pills, they would have been crushed up and flushed into my stomach tube. The prescription medicine for sepsis and/or pneumonia, however given, was not renewed. It was an empiric drug, one in which effectiveness is not proven through science, but through experiment and observation. I expect it had time limitations and had not been effective. Also, my prescribed sleeping medication was never renewed again. I was grossly sleep deprived. I asked a nurse one time "Isn't this what they do to war prisoners?"

The discharge sheet indicated a follow-up should be made with the facility's MD. Who? He was a fleeting fellow, coming and going sporadically suiting his own schedule. I saw him only once in the over seven months in which I resided in the nursing home, and that was many months after I had arrived. Everyone thought I was a lost cause, I expect. As it turned out, I wouldn't be.

"Tougher than old shoe leather," my mother would have said.

CNAville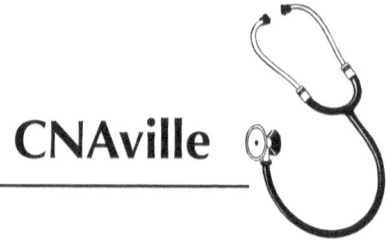

There are some people who are born to be caregivers. Often, they seek out work in nursing homes, assisted living facilities, or find employment with private nursing agencies. They are called CNAs, or certified nursing assistants. I was surrounded by them for quite a while and know those employed in the profession are extremely hard workers. It's not a job for the faint at heart, especially in a nursing home. If I found any CNA lacking in caretaking assistance, it appeared to be a matter arising from deficiencies in training or poor facility oversight rather than bad-apple individuals.

To become a CNA, an applicant does not need a high school diploma or GED unless under the age of 18. The training is short and inexpensive and can get the naturally born caretakers on the job quickly. I was very fortunate to have care from a few CNAs who were studying to become registered nurses and working in the nursing home for experience. Unfortunately, many healthcare training programs do not include hands-on encounters, a serious shortcoming in my opinion. Briefly, nursing home CNAs perform bathing and grooming, feeding and documenting intake, checking vitals, and minor wound care. They also move, turn, and transport patients and change linens.

One of my first interactions with a CNA could have resulted in an unfortunate mishap for the both of us. Somehow, though, the universe aligned to prevent it. The CNA was an older, stocky woman with years of experience, I'm sure. However, every new patient encounter and situation is different. As I had become not much more than a big wad of dough without a leavening starter, it was a tricky business to move me from bed, to feet, to wheelchair.

In a first attempt to get me up and going, she managed to prop me up into a wobbly standing position. But it went dangerously askew. I needed to be parallel to her body so she could guide me back and into the chair. We both became unbalanced. She kept saying "Step left, step left." I knew which foot was left, and I knew which way was left. However, there was no transmittal message to the brain for the movement. Finally, before we toppled together her adrenalized strength kicked in and the feat was accomplished. But not without an upset look on her face that I read as "Why didn't you just step left?"

Why indeed? In early conversations with our library's consumer health employee and follow-up with my own computer research, I found a hard blow to the head at the area where mine occurred could affect coordination of voluntary motor movement, balance, equilibrium, and muscle tone. Spot-on, I would say.

The chaotic nature found at times in a nursing home could have been partially mitigated by the posting of facility procedures for CNAs which should have been kept current. Caregivers need to have clear instructions from management about every nitty-gritty care process pertaining to job performance. They are owed this. Patients are owed this. I found the deficiency in both post-hospital care settings, the nursing home and in assisted living. Strangely enough, it was more so in assisted living. How difficult can it be to post directions and updates?

One problem was with the picking up of soiled clothing from your shared room in the nursing home. Clothes could be wet with urine, crusted with drips or drops of whatever, or otherwise dirtied by daily living. In my spartan room, a CNA would come in and put soiled clothing in the bottom drawer of the wardrobe where clean clothes were hung. She would tell me the clothing would be picked up by the morning CNA. This was not the morning CNA's understanding. And there the clothing remained until it was found some days later. Another CNA would hang dirtied clothing over my wheelchair. Still another once shoved it into a bureau drawer containing my books and other personal items. The issue could have been easily remedied by having proper instructions and procedures posted in a place where employees knew to look for them.

I can only assume that daily body washing procedures for bedded residents were not well taught in CNA training schools. Every day was a new adventure. Who's going to wash what? My face was always cleaned. Nice and refreshing. Usually, my upper chest and back were washed also. I would roll from side to side so a CNA could reach most of my back. One came and simply lightly washed over my clavicles. I thanked her and said, "This is the first time someone has just washed my clavicles." She just shyly smiled, maybe not familiar with the term. For the nappy wearers, hygiene was performed when the nappy was changed. I asked one CNA if she would wash my very short hair using the small plastic basin at bedside. She said no, simply NO! Perhaps a bad apple?

Recovery Expectations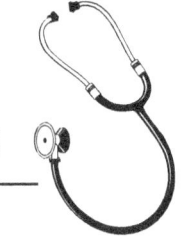

Both my daughters realized I was extremely ill. Neither really understood why. Nor could they imagine the impact the illness would have on my life. They were led to believe I had suffered an unfortunate cascade of serious, unrelated, and detrimental health events.

In the research stage of my healthcare odyssey, I called a Brain Injury Association of America representative to discuss medical diagnoses and the factors that play into making decisions. To my chagrin, I learned that a treatment plan might be initiated based on only one, or perhaps two symptoms. Consideration of a more complicated medical scenario when circumstances don't mesh is the road less taken. That seemed to fit my own case.

Now in a nursing home, I quickly realized there were two types of patients. Some were winding down to their last hurrah, and others were being propped up through physical and occupational therapy. Those receiving therapy after an injury or surgery would ultimately return home. I was in limbo land. Would I regain swallowing, muscular strength, balance, and motor ability? What would be my path, last hurrah or propping up? Would I ever have the chance to live independently again?

The facility's therapy room was large, well-staffed and equipped. Anne was impressed and envisioned me making good progress from therapeutic reprogramming and exercise. I was a disappointment to her. Two major health factors kept me in the slow lane. My degree of exhaustion resulting from the hospital debacle ranged in the -10 zone, unimaginable to others. A therapist would come to my bed at no scheduled time to wheel me to the therapy room and back to bed. Early on in my nursing home stay, a CNA told the therapist on return to my bed from a therapy session, "Oh no, she has to sit in the chair for a while." Strength building, I understood that. But I was not up to it yet. I sat in the wheelchair way too long waiting for what felt like a torturous ending of life. My daughter had my welfare at heart when urging me on with motivational jargon. But I felt like a failure. I had to gently let her know this tactic would not be helpful. While coaching may be a good strategy for young kids playing T-ball, it wasn't going to work for me. My mind/body connection was on its own timetable.

A second issue was lack of sleep, again in the -10 zone. I was taking sleep medication before I was hospitalized and continued during my hospital stay. The prescription would not be renewed until the nursing home's psychiatrist had his say. However, no psychiatrist was on board and there was never a renewal. Nighttime was often noisy long after midnight. Some doors had to be left open at night to rooms housing last hurrah patients.

The Puerto Rican woman in the adjacent bed was well on her way to a final breath, so our door was kept open at night. Noise from her side of the room, though, came during the day causing me equal opportunity noise anxiety. The woman's Puerto Rican daughter and son-in-law came daily to feed her a little lunch using sippy cup and spoon. "Abre la boca," they would shout. "Abre la boca." They shouted it again and again until she opened her mouth. The Spanish phrase for open your mouth became a part of my vocabulary. Then they yelled, "Swallow, swallow." Why in English, I didn't know. She would hold the food in her mouth, as dementia patients sometimes do, as swallowing is no longer automatic.

Occasionally, they asked a male Puerto Rican CNA to feed her, and he did the same with his booming male voice. "Abre la boca; swallow, swallow!" I had to remind him I was the co-occupant in the room and didn't appreciate his yelling. He quieted down a little. Much later, a young Puerto Rican woman said to me, "Puerto

Ricans are loud." A cultural or DNA thing? I came to realize my bedridden, last hurrah neighbor did have a bit of selective hearing.

The continuing nursing home cacophony and lack of sleep hindered my progress. Additionally, what I had later learned from the consumer health librarian perpetuated my belief that I had suffered a brain injury. She had accessed comments from a brain injury internet support group and read them to me. There were similar statements reflecting the overall sentiment that the brain's intake and processing ability becomes limited and skewed after injury. Halleluia! I was jubilant. I'm not crazy after all! That would explain why I tired so easily from a minimum of input, couldn't multi-task, needed televisions to be turned off, and just wanted to not be bothered.

Neurotic Neurons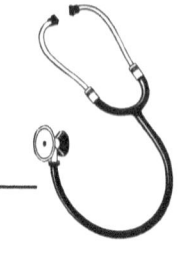

At this point in my nursing home stay, I still had no awareness of my hospital history. Only by looking back from where I am today can I make the following assessment. Whatever was happening with my body/brain connection fell well within the realm of the twilight zone. Critical analysis of the medical aspects of sepsis remnants pummeling a damaged brain would have been a daunting task. There was no one willing to take a leap and figure out cause and effect. I am not surprised, though, because records and reports were discordant enough to pummel any physician's brain.

The all around not-knowing syndrome crept into the nursing care facility as well. No discussions took place with me about my needs or wellbeing. My daughter was the only one to receive reports or information and passed it on to me. I had no opportunity for explanation or clarification, although it was apparent I was not cognitively impaired. I had the ability to think, question, understand, and respond.

Anne met with evaluation staffers early on who maintained I had refused to do this or had refused to do that. A misunderstanding evolved regarding physical therapy. Therapists would come to my room at any time of the day to take me to the therapy room. I would explain that I needed a nappy change. I did not want to end up in therapy doing exercise with urine running down my leg and onto the floor. They said, "Just switch on your call light." The therapists understood how things were done on their side of the workplace, but not on ours. I knew no one would be responding anytime soon and told them to just return to the therapy room. This happened maybe twice, and my comment was construed as pure refusal without a reason. Also, it seemed I wasn't reaching insurance-provider therapy goals. So sorry. One notable therapy event required me to use a walker to go from point A to point B, possibly a defined distance goal. The therapist would be alongside me with a steadying hand on the walker. This was boring stuff, and her mind was elsewhere. Her footwork was automatic. One step, another, then another. Suddenly my knees buckled, stopping me stone cold, and sending her toppling to the floor. Goal not met.

Another incongruous medical discovery was revealed after I had a high blood pressure reading. A medical technician was called for a bedside heart scan using a portable computer and scanning wand. My daughter came to update me – my heart was enlarged. What! Does this present a problem? She was told nothing else. At the same time, and unknown to me, my feet had been swelling. A CNA noticed and asked if anything was being done about it. This was the signal prompting that a diuretic, or "water pill," be added to the pill box.

Unfairly again, I was being accused of refusing to take a mucous buster treatment, a misted medication given through a mask with a tube connected to a noisy machine. I believe I was supposed to have treatments three times a day. What the situation boiled down to was that flurried day nurses, realizing that no treatment had been given, asked if I wanted to skip it. Sure, I did. It was a loud, no-remedy nuisance. More refusals were noted. The male night nurse's story about the mist treatment was more piqued as will be related in another chapter.

As a precursor to unknown skin perplexities throughout my many years' health adventure, the derma denizens were now making a first appearance. I had heard that a dermatologist visited the facility on rare occasions. I believe it was a philanthropic gesture. Unfortunately, I was never able to connect with her. One unnatural incident occurred one evening when my daughters were visiting. I demonstrated my version of skin exfoliation, in largesse, happening on the tops of my feet. I pulled at a small piece of loose skin which led to a good-sized patch peeling off. Soft, pink skin was underneath. My younger daughter looked at me in amazement and asked if I felt anything. I said no, "You have a go." There we were, taking turns, peeling and guffawing. What price laughter!

The medical mishmash presented in this narrative, although personal, does have a purpose. The shear extent of unharmonious body variables resulting in my distress demonstrated how brain signaling disruption through head injury can impact your life. In a healthy brain with about 10 million neurons firing constantly, how many of mine may have been firing in a haphazard fashion, or not at all. Just a blow to the back of my head evidenced by a four-inch laceration. Mighty powerful! And no one caught on.

Feeding Fiascos

I was on a phone call to my family in Bonita Springs, Florida, and speaking individually with each member. It was my teenage grandson's turn. As is typically the case, this age group temporarily exists on its own planet. He was unsure of what to say to an unwell grandmother, so I tried to liven up the conversation. It was time for my tube feeding. I joked with him and said they were bringing in my feed, which is how I referenced it. No response. Then I assured him, no it wasn't hay, or oats, or grass or anything like that, just liquid to be tubed into my stomach. He wasn't particularly amused and shortly retreated to his planet, thinking I must be on my own as well.

Daily feedings were seldom on schedule. Usually, I received four to five a day, sometimes the last at midnight. After entering the nursing home, it was a must to keep prescribed follow-up appointments as designated by the hospital, no matter your strength, endurance, or whether you had been fed. It was beneficial to be fed beforehand as transport and waiting times could run into a long stretch without nourishment. Feeding was about an hour-long process. I was on a tight schedule one day to keep a doctor's appointment. I asked the male nurse if he could speed it up. He showed me a small, plastic adjustor encircling the tube and said it could minimally change the flow. He was able to speed it up, and my daughter and I were off to the doctor. Another time, I asked a different nurse if she could do the same. She replied there was no way she could do that. I pointed to the little plastic gadget around the tube and asked if it was used to adjust flow. She seemed flustered then told me in no uncertain terms that I didn't know what I was talking about. Although the feeding process was slow, these were the only two times I asked to have it speeded up. I was not a pushy patient. For one appointment there was no time for one beforehand. The medical visit ran much longer than expected, so they rushed to feed me as soon as I had returned.

The manual feedings didn't go on for too long though, as the nutritionist decided I would do better with a slow, calibrated feeding. This would be delivered by an automatic pump. Nursing homes don't just have these on hand, so they ordered one. It came, was set up, and didn't work. Then another was ordered. My days of the pump's ear-deafening beep, beep, beeps now became the norm. It was the pump from hell and signaled with beeps when not pro-grammed properly. This was almost every day. It seemed appropriate that nurses would be trained to use it. I asked a nurse about it, and she replied, "If you've used one, you're good to go. They're all about the same." She soon learned the fallacy of her own words. No one seemed to be able to correctly program it, invariably setting off the beeps.

The new regime consisted of seventeen hours on the pump and seven hours off resulting in more time spent in bed. Supposedly, feeding was to start at 4:00 p.m. and end at 9:00 a.m. So much for that. Often a CNA would get me into bed at 4:00 p.m. to ready me for feeding. No nurse came. Two or so hours later the nurse ap-peared, punched in the code, and left. Ten to fifteen minutes later the obnoxious beeps started. She was so far down the hall by then, she couldn't hear the alarm. I had to endure loud beeps for up to twenty minutes until someone came for a retry. This could go on day or night, as an empty feeding bag was replaced throughout the seventeen hours.

Having feedings delayed held up daily routines when fortunate enough to even have one. The nurse whom I'd previously had a row with became upset about the whole new system and me having more in-bed time. I understood her viewpoint. In her heart she knew I had the best chance of leaving the nursing home alive and moving on than any other resident. Sometimes she angrily prodded me on to get with it. Then I became angry. I know now, they were good faith prods. Management recognized we weren't syncing and moved her to another section of the facility. Good call.

Another unfortunate situation arose from poor instructions given to CNAs about nappy changing while I was hooked up for feeding. Apparently, some just assumed they were not to disturb anything, afraid of causing a mishap. With so many hours in bed without a nappy change, you can imagine the urinary outcome. Everything was soaked around and under me in the morning. Fortunately, it didn't happen often. At times like this the wheat was separated from the chaff, staff wise. One CNA would gladly take me to shower, understanding my embarrassment and discomfort. Another would not, acting like the circumstances were my fault and only sponging me down at bedside. Of course, bedding had to be changed. That was a given.

To Taste or Not to Taste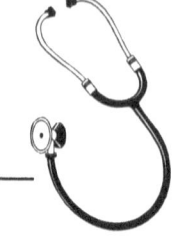

can empathize with covid survivors who temporarily lost their sense of taste. As an NPO patient, I, too, needed to taste. I missed the sensation. By happenstance, my daughters played into a taste testing adventure. My younger daughter had purchased medical cotton swabs online and had them sent to my daughter here in West Palm Beach. She often visited me and sometimes came with a soda or frosty shake. My mouth watered. It was time to share. She would dip a swab into the drink, and I would swipe it over my taste buds. A moment of pleasure. But when would my swallowing return?

The nursing home did have a speech therapist. In my case, her therapy was for swallowing. The two involve very similar methods. Fortunately, I was on board with insurance. Since I had no hospital memory, I didn't know what my hospital therapy entailed. The nursing home speech therapist would occasionally come to me at bedside, ask about my welfare, chat a little, and leave. I believe she tested me maybe two or three times with a teaspoon of water to see if I could swallow. I could not. After several months, the therapist told me she would be away for around six weeks as her husband was having out-of-state cancer treatments. Her replacement came and gave me a list of oral exercises, which she demonstrated. I was to do them daily. That's more like it, I thought.

Nevertheless, each day was dragging me down with a heightened sense of hopelessness. I was beginning to see no future for myself. The beep, beep, beeping of the feeding pump, the nappies, the nightly cacophony. They had also started me on a small, whirring respiratory machine with attached plastic mask to breathe in a medicated mist. The treatment was to relieve coughing with its ghastly sputum secretions. There was no remedy for that condition which still plagues me today. However, it did cause me strife with a male nurse who came in the middle of the night to set it up. I was supposed to have three treatments daily, but usually it boiled down to one at night. This turned into another patient refusal nightmare. He'd set me up and say "Don't touch anything until I get back." He'd be away for 15 to 20 minutes. When he got back, I'd have the mask off as well as the infernal whirring machine turned off. He'd unleash his fury at me, an ominous scolding. It became a ritual. Another nurse had told me the misted medication ran out long before even 10 minutes. I knew I had the right to refuse medical treatments, so I could have nixed it altogether.

You would have to think funny when things weren't especially so. Another male nurse, not one of the regulars, came one evening to set up the feeding system. He couldn't get the pouch of liquid to flow into the tube and tried at length; twisting, squeezing, turning the pouch this way and that. Suddenly, a burst of liquid sprayed everywhere, on my bed, my gown, his shirt, the floor, the venetian blinds on the window behind. Both of us in dismay. Brute force, the male way of doing things got the best of him but didn't accomplish the task.

My biggest disappointment in the nursing home happened one morning when I saw my wheelchair had gone missing. I asked a CNA about it. "Oh, they may be cleaning it," she said in a no worries manner. The facility owned the chair but a savvy physical therapist who knew her way around ambulatory equipment had fitted it to suit me. My trusted prosthesis was not returned, and its replacement was sub-par. With more and more demoralization, I became caught in an undertow.

I now let my daughter know I saw no future for myself and wanted to discontinue feedings. She put forth a scenario that I'd get weaker, they would send me back to the hospital; I'd get better, they would send me back to the nursing home. Back and forth, ad infinitum. All so gruesome sounding. That put me off for a couple of days. Really, I no longer cared to live with unrelenting misery and no end in sight. I notified each nurse attending me that I wanted no more feedings. This went against their professional beliefs, and for many against their religious beliefs. They were upset and had not been advised about what to do. One came stealthily at night and hooked me up to a bag of liquid. I let her know she was not to go against my wishes. Sweetly, she said she just wanted me to have a little nutrition. Another came all flustered, not knowing what to do about medications. She asked if I was supposed to have them. "I don't think so," I said.

On the fourth day without nutrition, the nursing home's risk management employee came to talk with me about my decision without taking a proselytizing stance. She did say something to the effect that if she were me, she would feel the same way. The validation was appreciated, but I recognized she couldn't say "Do the same thing," even if it were true. On the fifth day, two higher level staff members came to my bedside asking if I would be amenable to having a mobile van come in, equipped with testing equipment and medical personnel, to evaluate my swallowing. Who knew there were such mobile labs? Yes, I was amenable. Bring it on.

Cookie Mayday

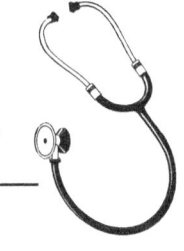

A testing van for swallowing evaluation arrived at my facility the day after I had given consent. It parked at the exit door near my room, and I was wheeled out and up the van's ramp, then positioned under an overhead recording monitor. A tray of small plastic cups was placed across my wheelchair armrests. I'm not sure of the method used to transmit views of throat swallowing to the monitor, but knew as a designated NPO patient it certainly didn't involve drinking thick, chalky barium as some testing requires.

The plastic cups were lined up in a row in a progression of consistencies and textures from easy to swallow, to more difficult. I started with a sip of water. One sip went down, no coughing, no spitting. Then the second was swallowed. Oh, happy day! Viewing and note taking in elongated medispeak took several minutes between each test. Milk came next. Tasted good. I passed. Pudding, applesauce, I was on a roll. The final clincher was broken bits of a chocolate chip cookie. I chewed; I swallowed. Double happy day! The therapist wheeled me back to the bathroom sink in my room saying, "Brush." Thinking now that I had eaten, it was necessary to brush my teeth. I made a comment to that effect. "Oh, no," she stammered, "You should have been brushing all along." That was a revelation. I learned from her that oral care was needed while NPO. Bacteria in the mouth could lead to bacteria growth in the lung when swallowing saliva, she told me. Up to this point, I had rarely been given the opportunity to brush my teeth at bedside.

Word was quick to get around the nursing home that my swallowing function was up and running. Proper messaging had returned. Some nurses were so elated they immediately removed the

NPO classification from their computers but were then told to re-enter it. The change had to travel through the kingdom of all things official. Soon after the testing, the regular therapist returned. Gossip got back to me that some of her workmates in the therapy department had chastised her for giving me insufficient testing and care.

The facility was fortunate to have an excellent nutritionist on staff who decided I would continue to have a small, nightly tube feeding while the transition to solid food took place. My meals were mostly pureed. I decided, overall, they were tasty and satisfying, although I couldn't always distinguish what meat I was eating. Then I moved on to mechanicals. I imagine the term came about because food items are manually chopped, or shredded into small pieces by using kitchen hand tools.

A couple of oddities occurred after I had become an eater. I hadn't given much thought to my wrist with its two encircling plastic bands. The one designating my NPO status had been removed. But the other, what was that? Finally, I asked. They told me it signified my liquids had to be thickened. Simultaneously, I could not have anything by mouth, but liquid intake by mouth had to be thickened? Both bands had been around my wrist since my arrival No one had ever questioned the anomaly. I asked to have the remaining band removed but it only caused confusion in the kingdom, so I let it go.

The second off-the-wall encounter involved the absentee doctor who had never peeked in on me before. He knew I was now eating and had concerns about tube removal. He wanted to have a look at the tube. As it had been surgically placed, he seemed unsure of the method for removal. We weren't to that point yet, as everything had to be funneled through the nutritionist. As he left my room, the doctor inquired about my welfare. As usual, my issue was inability to sleep, and I told him that. He said he would look into it. I never saw or heard from him again.

Once the day came to remove the tube, staff came to get me from the physical therapy room. I was told to lie down on my bed and remain there for one hour after they, yes, just physically yanked it out. About a year later I received a bill for the procedure, over eight hundred dollars. I had progressed to assisted living and was handling most of my affairs. I called the company and said, "You must have used an incorrect medical code on this bill." He said it was correct. The same code is used for surgically placing the tube and then manually pulling it out. Then he asked about my insurance. I named the company and added it was specifically for nursing home patients. Then he said, "Forget it. You don't owe anything." I asked why the bill had been so delayed. "We were being audited."

Goodbyes in Order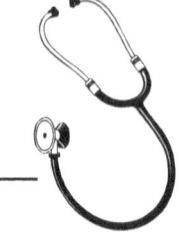

A nursing home stay in your own or your family's life is very possible. There were 1.2 million residents in 15,000 certified nursing homes in 2022, either for short-term medical incidents requiring physical rehabilitation, or a long-term stay for a chronic disease that results in death. Around 70% of the facilities are for-profit businesses. The remainder are government, religious, or non-secular entities.

Before I left the hospital, I was asked to choose a nursing home from a list of about twelve. This was at a time when my memory was returning. While to my knowledge I was rarely asked anything in the hospital, staff handling my transition let me make a choice for next-step placement. My daughter was not asked to be there, and I had no knowledge of existing facilities. I narrowed my choice to three, based on distance between my daughter's home and the nursing home. Then I narrowed it to one. The appropriate procedure would have been to let my daughter research the three. She could have given recommendations before I had to choose. The process seemed to be a quick encounter just to keep the ball rolling.

Although I've mentioned untoward events in my nursing home stay, none were of a malicious nature. Shortcomings seemed to have resulted from inadequate managerial oversight and lack of communication with staff about present and changing procedures. These facilities house the most vulnerable of our population. I must credit my facility for having been fully engaged in providing activities and entertainment to divert residents from painstaking daily routines. Many were wheeled into a recreational area by CNAs who remained there to wheel them back. If there was musical entertainment, many

CNAs would not hesitate to put forth their best dance moves. What I am left with are some poignant memories of staff and residents that blur most sentiments of negativity. Some of these are acknowledged here.

One tall, male CNA studying to become a nurse was so ecstatic after the NPO status change, he asked if I would like a drink of water." Of course," I said. Off he went. He was gone for a while. When he returned, he offered me a large-sized, Styrofoam cup with a straw poking out from its lid. I took a sip. It was not plain water, and I joyfully exclaimed, "It's lemon flavored!" A few staff gathered at bedside were wondering where he got the flavoring. Wherever it came from was of no concern to me. He had made an excellent decision.

When my granddaughter was visiting and it was feeding time, a male nurse asked if she would like to watch. I wondered what she'd say, as in the past the sight of blood had made her feel faint to the point of passing out. There would be no blood, so she told the nurse she was on board to watch. It was a short process, but this small act effectively infused the three of us with a grand sense of sharing.

Two close-to-retirement, but awesomely strong ladies were charged with weighing residents. They were experts. On one of my urine-soaked mornings, they came to my bed to weigh me. I indicated my situation. No problem. They were totally in control of this type of unsettling event. They grabbed the bedding under me using it as a gurney and deftly transferred me to the weighing bed. As I was wondering about weight accuracy, they assured me the weight of wet bedding would be subtracted from the total weight. They were incredible caregivers.

Lucious lips, as I had become to think of her, was a single woman with two older children. She had been seeing someone as a romantic interest. One night there was a knock, knock, knocking at the glass entrance door. Someone on staff yelled to her, "There's somebody at the door asking for you." I overheard the conversation as it was taking place. He was imploring her to just up and run away with him. Begging her, in fact. Enchanted by those luscious lips, he was. But she, of course, knew he was a lovesick puppy and assured him she could do no such thing.

Some of the concourse people thoroughly enchanted me. They were the mentally waning residents who spent a good amount of time wheeling around the rectangular-shaped walkway which I had come to call the concourse. They had lots of gusto and spent a good amount of their day wheeling around on it, as I did occasionally for exercise. One woman would invariably stop at the corner of one wheelway when she saw a certain stylized painting on the wall above her. It was the torso of a person holding up a hand with fingers extended. She would then hold up her hand, fingers extended, and count one, two, three, four, five.

At last, after 9 months it had come time for me to make an upward move toward wellness and independence. I had made enough progress to qualify for assisted living, a whole new adventure. A few staffers came to say they were happy to see me go, then qualified that with "Not because we don't like you." They were overly delighted when someone was able to leave alive instead of under a white sheet, which was the common occurrence.

III

ASSISTED living

AL Here I Come

My two daughters had scouted out four or so local assisted living (AL) facilities and brought me brochures and other marketing information to look over. It was my decision about where I would go, and it was difficult to choose as I couldn't visit the facilities myself. After looking over the material, we had a question-and-answer session. They left the brochures with me, and I was to call if I had more questions.

I chose an AL facility located halfway between my daughter Anne's home and her workplace, a nice bonus. I was a bit leery of its size: five, six-story buildings in a semi-circle. I had never lived in any type of large, multi-story apartment complex before and wondered how easy it would be to make friends. As it turned out, only one building was for AL residents. The other four were for independent living residents. The AL activity calendar finally sold me. It listed a variety of events and had an exercise class for those who were wheelchair bound.

I had my own apartment on the 6th floor. Anne had chosen it with the thought that I would enjoy the pool view. Plus, I would see the sunset every night. She was right. It suited me well. She selected the furniture and accessories from my townhouse and called for movers to deliver it. I gave her carte blanche authority to call the shots for its arrangement but for one, "Put the recliner directly across from the television for optimal viewing." Not that I had ever watched it much, but probably would now. A couple of days later my daughter Laura and family came to hang my many special pictures and attractive wall décor. I should be happy here, right?

The facility provided on-site benefits including doctors, physical therapy, and transportation to medical appointments within a 10-mile radius. I would take advantage of it all. I just wanted everything to be easy for everyone. After settling in, I met with the AL director to discuss care plans. Needs are based on care levels, the greater the need the higher the cost, of course. I was ready to divest myself from the food requirement of mechanicals and take on medication management on my own. As mentioned previously, the food preparation technique termed mechanicals consists of cutting up harder to chew foods, mostly meats, into small pieces. For example, if I was served a hamburger at the nursing home, the meat would have been crumbled up inside the bun with the soft bun left intact.

The decision was made in the nursing home to have the AL doctor give approval for changes. The facility was in between doctors at the time, so my requests went unheeded. I had to wait for a new doctor to come on board. Mechanicals it was then, but nobody paid attention. No one informed food staff of the preparation process. On came the regular food. Did I complain? Absolutely not! I knew I was able to chew and swallow. In a few weeks a light-bulb moment came on in the AL director's head. "Gail is not getting mechanicals!" The following evening, a plate of food was set down in front of me. Thirty seconds later kitchen staff rushed to snatch it back up saying, "We'll be right back." The plate of food was redelivered. All food was cut up, no matter its original consistency. The pieces of a dinner roll would be tossed to our resident ducks.

Speaking of kitchen and food service, everything about it was slow and haphazard. CNAs helped with dining room service which I imagine reduced staffing costs. Really, only a few CNAs who paid attention to resident needs would have sufficed. One visually impaired woman came daily to eat. She needed her chair pulled out to sit in, then needed to be pushed up to the table. Once she was in the chair, the CNA invariably trotted off before pushing her in. She had to call for help again. She also needed someone to help cut up her food, which was most of the time. The warm meal was on its way to cold before anyone came. Where was the assisted living?

Before getting approval for handling medicines on my own, CNAs with med tech training brought my pills and watched me gulp them down. A few times, a CNA would bring me one pill when I was supposed to have two of that same one. I would point this out. She had to go to the medicine cart in the hallway, check it out, and bring me the second one.

At last, a new contracted doctor came aboard. I had no idea of the background given to him about my condition and what led me to assisted care. And I will never know. Again, medical records had either gone by the wayside, or not been referenced. I wheelchaired into the doctor's on-site office for a first meeting. He could tell I was not cognitively impaired, so he granted my two requests. An unfortunate situation occurred later in our patient relationship when he hired a new physician's assistant. She wasn't up to par and interfered with my prescription routine. She was told, and it should have been on record that I managed my own medicine. She messed up horribly with the prescription provider, and I was left to clean up the mess. Sometimes I thought she was mixing up patients. The overseeing physician may have been new in his profession and not thought that oversight was needed for his staff. Poor medical assistants and office managers can make or break a physician's business, and I finally had to call it quits with their unsatisfactory practice.

Time to Play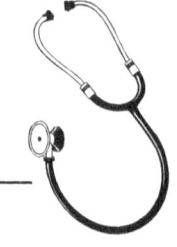

There was a much-admired activity director in AL who had been in that position for well over 10 years. He was one of a kind – compassionate, creative, smart, and all in. I assumed he had a heady budget as evidenced by all that was offered for residents. Bells, whistles, and more. Any book about elders will say they need mental and physical stimulation, plus social interaction. Tell that to the 80% or so of the residents who didn't want to come out and play. They weren't buying it. Only a few social events such as special occasion parties would draw them in. Then, too, I knew a few who played cards in a foursome once a week with three others mostly from independent living. Perhaps this once-a-week activity was all they needed.

Based on my experience in AL, I will digress by giving my take on the often-meager showing at daily activities. I'm sure there are admittance criteria for accepting residents in the different kinds of care facilities. I know I was evaluated before I moved from the nursing home to this step-up style of living. Little did I know this complex was part of a publicly traded corporate entity of which there were 140 or more in twenty-seven states. Their bottom line, of course, was renting rooms. I could see that criteria had been stretched to keep apartments filled. I would term these apartment fillers as the Half ways. Halfway to nursing home care, halfway to dementia care. Then there were those just waiting for God, so to speak. If a resident needed additional care and attention than what AL could provide, they paid for private service providers to come in and help them. I inquired once about using volunteers to assist with motivating individuals and getting them to the activity room. Nope. Liability issue. Having numerous Half ways in our building defeated the very essence and intent of assisted living. However incongruous care facilities are, though, the need is there. Residents should be offered all that is promised and paying for whether they participate or not.

As mentioned, the calendar of events was a draw for me. I imagined myself being able to give it all a go. I did, to a degree. As a resident with unacknowledged and unknown medical disabilities, I didn't know what to expect health wise. One day early on in my residency, I had to flee the activity room. There was a fog over me, my vision went haywire, and I said I needed to go to the ladies room. I motored my way out of the activity room in my wheelchair using hand and foot propulsion. The ladies room was close by, but a very busy-patterned carpet lay between one room and the other. Looking down at the carpet made me nauseous, and my left foot was amiss with its motor task. Making a long story short, I ended up wedged between the toilet and sink, against the wall, and was unable to get into my wheelchair. Funny now, but scary then.

There was an emergency pull string. I used it. It was positioned to be pulled straight down, but I think my sideways pull didn't register. No one came. Residents do wear wristbands to call someone; however, in my anxious state I had a mental failure. Then I mustered up whatever ability was needed to get me out of the predicament, exit the room, and call a CNA to push me to my apartment saying I felt dizzy.

Sometimes when I engaged in a modified chair activity called Zumba requiring quick thinking and movement, my brain became flummoxed, and I had to stop. I was the baby there in AL. Why couldn't I keep up with others who were much older. At times I felt I was running on fumes only. Towards the end of a longer activity I would say "My buzzer went off," meaning no more. I had to imme-diately go to my room and lie down.

During Covid-19 lockdown, essential-worker activity leaders showed us what they were made of. Daily, they came to each door with their "lift your spirits" cart and a mindset to match. One day a week they brought ice cream, another day they came with snacks. And for liquid spirit consumers, they would come bearing red or white wine once a week. There were puzzle and activity books to loan. Sometimes they played music in the hallways or had games where you could sit in your doorway and participate. Once-in-awhile they came costumed to reflect a theme, probably orchestrated by the corporate entity. This was a truly AL inspired respite during lockdown.

About a month into lockdown, though, our AL residents received a well-written memo from our community's food services director. Their considerate staff would be bringing around a daily "lift your spirits" cart. Well, duh! Thank you, but this is already going on here in AL. This was a perfect example of the constant, no overall management syndrome present in the facility, Covid-19 or no Covid-19. We were supposed to be one community under one roof, but it didn't work that way. Although we were wrinkled, we didn't expect that to be the case in our care environment. Smooth and easy living was seldom the case.

Who's in My Shoes

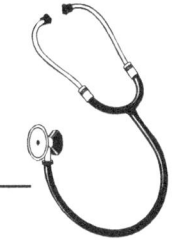

Never having had a medical diagnosis of brain injury while in the hospital, I was hesitant to use the term when talking to others about events leading to assisted living. An implied courtesy existed to refrain from being too nosey, so I didn't get many questions. As it turned out, though, there were two residents in the facility who already knew me. They had lived in the small, townhouse community where I had lived. They wanted the scoop, so I obliged. I told the story as I knew it at the time, a mixture of facts intertwined with pieces from my fabricated memories. Never did I use the term traumatic brain injury or severe sepsis. Still, I received their "poor thing" sentiments, and that was that.

It wasn't long before I realized a body/mind remake was occurring. Starting with the body, mine was talking to me. Many discomforts and minor medical symptoms were plaguing me, and I was unable to pinpoint whether anything really warranted medical attention. I did learn later from a brain injury publication that indeed this can happen. These were not hypochondrial occurrences. A psychiatrist who periodically came to the facility saw me as a patient a few times. I reluctantly postured to her in a roundabout way that perhaps faulty brain messages were having their way with me, physically. Her body language and succinct reiteration of what she thought I was saying told me I should just drop it. Everything about me was not making sense.

I also talked to a psychotherapist about my continual discomforts. One example was occasional tightening and pain at the end of the breastbone. Off to the doctor most people would have run, maybe thinking it was a heart-related symptom. Scary heart stuff!

But I was beginning to recognize brain dynamics. That's when I latched onto the descriptor "bogus." It became a repeated word in my vocabulary when doing battle with these bodily disturbances. Sometimes they came in rounds: head pain, shoulder tension, knife-like stab in the leg. I would say over and over, "It's bogus, means nothing, go away," or words to that effect always emphasizing the word bogus. Referring to my hospitalization, I used a three-word chant, "It's over, be happy, be well," to center and calm me. The therapist was complimentary about my tactics, and they worked for me.

Other extremely curious and oddball sensations came over me. One came from my pacemaker implant. Basically, a pacemaker is a battery with one or two wire leads to stimulate a slow heart rhythm with an electrical pulse. In the over 20 years that I've had one, I felt nothing. It was a silent partner doing its job of heartbeat regulation as needed. Then at about 10 months into my AL stay, I began to feel indescribable, annoyingly weird stimuli at the entry point where the wire leads attach to the battery. Also, I felt pulsing, sometimes in one side of the vein or in the other, especially where the wires are attached and threaded into the vein. On the left side, I would have to reposition my arm in bed at night so I wouldn't feel the pulsing with its unwanted sensations.

Another experience was seeing flashes of light with my eyes closed when I was in bed at night. When I opened my eyes, the left one was fuzzed over. Then it slowly cleared. These manifestations were thankfully short lived. Although they were unusual and very personal, I am again risking the "crazy" label to share them. Like myself, brain injured people may not have had access to a support group or sufficient information about their condition. I had to re-assure myself I couldn't be the only one experiencing unheard of oddities. Unfortunately, brain injury recovery cannot be quantified. It may be two steps forward and one back, seemingly only a minus-cule gain at a time. Frustrating remnants of injury may likely last a lifetime.

Personality wise, I began to interact with people differently. I was a speak when spoken to, answer when asked person. Quiet and reserved. Then I gradually evolved into a Chatty Cathy, like the more than half-century old doll by that name. Pull her string and off she went – blah, blah, blah. I had to remind myself to shut up when I noticed people's attention waning. I also developed a little chuckle like my aunt's. I uttered it after saying something, just as she had done, not that anything I had said was so funny. It was not often that I chuckled and never at an inappropriate time. Published materials from the Brain Injury Association of America say unsuitable behaviors may surface from brain injury and may need specialty treatment.

Cognitively speaking, I found I was remembering names, dates, and situational specifics better. My analytical and problem-solving skills were mostly on target, although slow. My self-assessment became a realization of slow, body/mind mending knotted with slow, body/mind ageing. This brought to mind a Marvin Gaye song lyric, "What's going on, what's going on." That, too, became another of my silly characteristics. I would hear someone speak a few words and immediately it would trigger a song reflecting those sentiments. Out of my mouth it would come, just as in the song. And I was never a musical person as far as singing goes.

Trauma Drama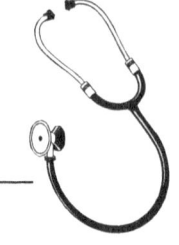

About a year and a half into my assisted living tenure and before I had begun my book writing mission, I had a tumultuous meltdown. Sensing the unknown trauma had brought on memory loss, my mind seemed to be stumbling through the black hole to find an exit. After learning the amnesia covered the entire hospitalization of twenty-six days, not just the thirteen that I had been recounting in my confused storytelling, it seemed a new truth was trying to surface.

Combine that revelation with relentless lack of sleep and there was bound to be a backlash. I began "acting out," the phrase often used to describe a child's wayward behavior when under duress. I expect the term is applicable to adults as well, but we try to tamp everything down to keep our psychological pain under wraps. I was irritable, sometimes short with people. I wanted to wheelchair down the hall and scream. I talked to myself in the closet about my state of mind. Then, an alarming occurrence triggered a mental shake up.

The situation happened one morning as I was approaching the elevator to go down to the first floor for an activity. I felt anxiety, along with hostility. Where was that coming from? The elevators were old and slow, but one was on its way. I'll be okay. The elevator is coming. Just get in it. You're okay. Unexpectedly, thoughts of hurting someone overtook me. Just get in the elevator. You'll be all right. What would I use as a weapon? A stick? A rock? I was not all right. Quickly, I returned to my apartment. I had to somehow reboot and refresh the screen.

I phoned my daughter Anne, asking her to come over as soon as possible. I tried not to voice neediness, but the ASAP reverberated and gave me away. She was grocery shopping and would come by when finished. That was a relief. When she arrived, I didn't go into details but just told her I was ready for her to spill. What she knew about my hospitalization, I needed to know. She said my kidneys were failing soon after I was hospitalized. Really? Serious stuff! I was shocked. But a rather quick reversal to the diagnosis followed as I later found out from my medical records. Dialysis or a kidney transplant seemed not to be on the horizon. The new worry was pneumonia. A doctor discussed my condition with her saying standard antibiotics weren't working. He had been apprehensive about prescribing the empiric drug mentioned earlier, the one for pneumonia, sepsis, and other treatment-resistant bacterial illnesses. Unknown to her, I was on a ventilator for a short stint as was later indicated by my records.

Then, after relating bladder issues to me and saying a doctor had told her my bladder had been perforated, she asked how I was holding up with the reveal of this information. It wasn't quite sinking in yet, but I assured her I would call the contracted, assisted living psychiatrist, if needed. Then I phoned my Bonita Springs' daughter, Laura, to give her an update. She reiterated again how hard it was to get questions answered in the hospital which left her frustrated and confused.

I decided to call the psychiatrist. She came to my apartment, and I told her of my acting out experiences and need to know mindset. She also had not known the specifics of my downfall, or I suppose it would be fall down, but then who did? We questioned how I might process the reveal, and I agreed to contact her if a maelstrom erupted.

The tumultuous meltdown did come. Nights of tossing and turning left me more washed out during the day than ever. Sometimes I mumbled or yelped during dozes. I remember a few of my out loud, apprehensive pleas, "No more pain; I can't take it anymore." Instinctively, I realized I was on my own. My brain was making a tsunamic-like attempt to change its landscape. In time, I was able to have longer and more restful sleeps. Healing.

I remember saying to the psychiatrist on one visit that I didn't envy her profession as the mind is essentially unknowable. And I still believe it.

Bookend Transgressions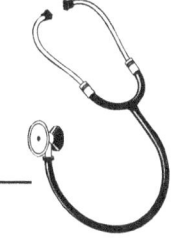

As a resident in assisted living, I felt confident I would receive CNA help as needed, be safe, and be respected. Wrong on all counts. I experienced five serious transgressions during my over three-year residency in the facility. The bookend wrongdoings, involving Medicare fraud, occurred at the beginning and the end of my stay. Sandwiched in between were three breaches of good conduct by managers consisting of deceit, cover-up, and flagrant disrespect.

The first Medicare fraud case was a particularly egregious act, set off by the lowest of the low. Fraud schemers working with facility insiders accessed my records and stole my Medicare insurance and social security numbers, plus the name of the facility doctor whom I was using as my primary care physician.

Here's how it worked. One day there was a knock at my door. I yelled, "Come in," as those of us with mobility issues do. I had been assured this was a safe and open environment with no daytime door locking needed. In came a woman with a well- conceived spiel about how the state had decided the elderly might be fearful of hurricanes and may need supportive counseling. Hurricane Irma had pounded the area the prior year. I thought perhaps the state government had been given grant money and everyone here was in the know about the visits. How easily we are deceived.

She asked me a few questions relating to hurricane situations, and I told her I had been through plenty. Seeing several books in my living area, she zeroed in on book talk. Then she dug into her bag and pulled out a business card, hers I assumed, to write a library internet address on the back which I could use to download books to an electronic device. I put the card aside, as I had no electronic device. If it was her business card, it should have been presented up front. Less than 15 minutes later, she left saying she would return in a month. She did. More book talk. When she showed up again, I began to get suspicious and told her I had to go to lunch.

Then came my Medicare summary statement. The jig was up. Payments had been made to a Ft. Lauderdale, Florida firm for one-hour psychotherapy services. I had been used, violated, and was extremely angry. The executive director at that time heard my story and said he would investigate it. I heard nothing back from him, ever. Not being one to just look the other way, I called Medicare fraud. Their answer, "We can't process it as fraud because you let her in."

The second fraud involved a private nursing guild with a contractual business arrangement with the facility. These can be beneficial, but their connection should be made transparent. You need to know who is walking into your room, why, and who is paying their salary. In two separate Medicare summaries I received, the private nursing agency billed Medicare for payment of eight skilled nursing visits which never happened, nor were they requested. These first claims were denied by Medicare. Then a third came showing a payment of over $1,200 made for another eight skilled nursing visits which never took place.

Ultimately, I had rounds with the nursing agency's manager who, in effect, was calling me a liar, as she insisted I did have the services. I got Medicare fraud involved again. They felt the fraud claim deserved investigation. As I wanted to report an outcome for this book, I called Medicare fraud to get an update. I was told it could take years for a resolution, or there might never be one. In my case, I'm sure there will never be one, as a high-level manager in AL was also an administrator for the nursing agency. Hand in hand, you see. She was asked to come to my apartment to discuss the matter, but never showed up. Very shortly thereafter, she resigned and moved out of state. (Circumstantial, of course.)

For those not Medicare initiated, sometimes a healthcare provider will choose not to pass on Medicare's twenty percent copay to the client. As clients receive no bill from the provider, they may throw the quarterly Medicare notices out thinking all is well. These summaries need to be scrutinized, and suspicion of fraud reported to the agency. I did my part.

Dustgate Conspiracy

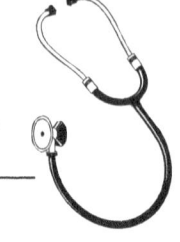

C ovid-19 was at bay leading toward complete lockdown in AL. Only residents, essential workers, and screened personnel for emergency needs would be allowed in. Meals were delivered and temperature and oxygen readings taken daily. It was quiet, and I felt safe from the outside world. But inside my apartment something bizarre was revving up. Since my medical trauma, I questioned every oddity. Are these occurrences real? Or is it me. Am I no longer quite right?

After showering one morning with a CNA's help, I picked up my hand mirror to reflect the back of my head in the mirror over the sink. It was a random action. But why today? A pink patch of scalp peeked back at me. Hair loss? Rubbing my fingers over the area, I felt flattened cowlicks whirled around the patch, as though they had been plastered there with glue. No amount of combing, smoothing, or grooming technique could coerce them into place. So, I became a bandana wearer, preserving my pride, of course.

Other strange incidents manifested at the same time, further casting a shadow over my reasoning. Waking one morning, I felt something stuck to my lower lip. Small and hard. I removed it and put it aside to examine after breakfast. You eat. You brush. A few brushes into it, I realized something gritty was in my mouth. I spit. Out with the toothpaste came what seemed to be beige insect egg cases. More of the tiny things were wedged between the toothbrush bristles. With disgust, I washed them out and flushed everything down the sink. Bad move. I should have saved them. Still, the lip specimen remained on the bathroom counter.

Also, excess dust was collecting on the floor at bedside, around my upholstered, ribbed-clothed recliner, and in wheelchair tracks. White dots appeared there also. Infestation? I sensed something was in and under my skin. Very unpleasant. Covid-19 was proliferating, so maybe it was a fecund time for who knows what else. Living on the top floor with a bathroom air vent opening to the crawl space under the roof, and bird nesting going on up there, I had to ponder the possible entry of tiny, unwanted trespassers.

I called the AL director, who was also a registered nurse, to advise me. No response. I called facility staff to have an apartment inspection or have the contracted exterminator come in. No response. Late on a Friday afternoon, well over a week and a half with no one paying attention, I called my daughter to air my aggravation. She inquired whether I might like to contact a regulatory agency. I was reluctant. People were dying during the pandemic. How big a deal was this? But I was paying a hefty sum for assisted living and getting unassisted living. Finally, becoming more distressed, I called the Agency for Healthcare Administration (AHCA). They listened to my rambling grievances and asked if I had called the Florida Ombudsman. "No, do I have to tell this story again?"

"Yes," was their reply, so I called on Monday spending a troublesome weekend of woe is me.

Prompted by the AHCA report, the AL director asked the facility manager to arrange an inspection. I told her I had previously called him myself with no response. An exterminator came with a canister and an attached spray hose, and the CNA accompanying him told me I had to leave the room for a few hours. "What are you spraying for?" I asked the exterminator. "You don't even know what's in here." I told my story and showed him the tiny specimens I had collected and placed on a black cloth. The lip specimen was there. He looked at them with his naked eye, was highly dubious, and mumbled he'd return the next day. Back he came the following morning with a cluster of sticky-bottomed paper boxes. These were placed here and there at his discretion. If the so-called infestation was parasitic, the offenders were not going to leave me for a sticky box, were they? After peeking into the boxes much later that day and seeing nothing, I collected them and scattered my specimens over their sticky bottoms. The exterminator returned the following morning. Seeing the boxes all together on the floor, he became furious. I explained my reasoning. He didn't want to hear it and angrily barked, "I have 15 years in the business and know what I'm doing!" He picked the boxes up along with a large fluff of dust in a plastic bag that I had provided. Perhaps the dust might hold a clue, I thought. I learned later when he had passed the AL director's door on the way out, she had called out to him asking if he had found anything. "It's just dust," he replied, holding up the bag.

Finally, I asked to go to the ER. Something was amiss, skin-wise. A small, medic's ambulance came with no to-do. I had asked that no spectacle be made. In the ER I was quickly diagnosed with lice, adult, acute. Back in my apartment, three applications of pesticide cream were lavished over my body on three consecutive nights, a distasteful procedure. Subsequently, I phoned the executive director (ED) about the diagnosis. He was in disbelief remarking, "This kind of thing never happens here." Then thinking of the commonly spread head lice he stammered, "Well, isn't it just a matter of shampoos and lotions?"

"No," I said. "It's not head lice."

He retorted that the facility manager had shown him the bag and told him, "It's all clear. It was just dust." I mentioned the specimen boxes to the ED. What did they show? He would get back to me, but never did.

The AHCA and Ombudsman both had my infestation story on record, but with Covid-19 on rampage there would be no mediation process anytime soon. That threw me into a new role – super sleuth. I needed answers and explanations. No one in AL would take on my cause, and I understood. I'm no dummy.

The issue of what happened to the specimen boxes remained. I surmised the pest control technician had disposed of them. Proof, I needed proof. I knew the company's name, but several branches were in West Palm Beach. To get the number of the branch serving us, I made scads of one-dollar calls to the 411-information line. Remember, I had no computer in my apartment. I started with a pleasant chat with the receptionist. She understood my dilemma and was more than willing to help me. The word lice just sets peoples' teeth on edge. Two calls later it became apparent receptionists had been instructed to tell me to call our facility manager. I already had. No response. We were stalled.

At my age and with a lifetime of experience behind me, it was time to play their game. A threat was now in order. I told the pest company's receptionist I might have a good lice story warranting media attention. Quickly she put me on hold, then came back with a message from the manager. It was a Friday, and he would call me the following Monday at noon. On Monday, I sat by the phone at the specified time. No call. Ten minutes went by, then fifteen. Then I called the company branch asking for the manager. He picked up the phone and seemed bewildered, as though he hadn't worked out a plausible story. Then he said the director and facility manager had just left his office and would shortly be over to see me. Now we're getting somewhere. They never showed up.

The whole lice ordeal lasted many months. I was sick and tired of dealing with it. Health conditions also loosely described as "sick and tired" double-downed on me. I was in touch with my daughter throughout the fiasco, and I would mention just dropping the case. When she asked how I was, I'd reply, "Sad." It was inconceivable that my life had come to this.

Wanting it to be over, I called the two state entities and said I would like to drop the case, expressing my opinion it would result in excuses and innuendo only. Then I wrote a letter to the executive director holding him and the facility manager accountable for poor judgment, lack of sensitivity and respect, and having no protocol in place for a report of infestation. In fact, the ER doctor who had replied to a nurse asking what facility I was from stated, "They should have handled it there." I attached all my invoices requiring cost payments associated with the incident totaling almost $400 and asked for reimbursement. No response. I called my attorney. Her take on the matter was it's a large corporation, all lawyered up, so you can kiss that money goodbye.

As to how lice found me during Covid lockdown, circumstances led me to believe it was from baby bear, sitting in my chair, and finding it just right. (*Goldilocks and the Three Bears.*) Around 2:00 a.m. one night I awoke and thought I might get a drink from the kitchen. I wheelchaired out the bedroom door, which I never fully shut at night, and made no noise. It was dark, but across the room there seemed to be someone fully reclining in my comfortable, nubbed fabric chair. I refocused. Yes, someone was there. She was highly engaged with her phone or small electronic device, then sensed my presence and stuttered, "I...I was just check...checking on you." Up she bolted and ran out the door leaving her hand-held radio transmitter by the chair Not knowing what to do with it, I finally decided to put it in the hallway outside my door where it ultimately would be picked up. To note, CNAs do check on residents at night, a quick in and out, unless a no entry sign is posted. My no entry at night sign went up immediately, along with an employee incident report.

Smoke But No Fire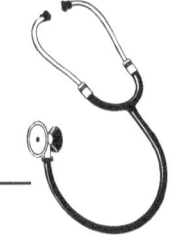

A n ongoing ruckus in my six-story building involved fire alerts
and so-called standardized procedures for evacuation. The
issue continued to exist for the entire three years I had resided there.
In a real fire, elevators cease operation, and sprinklers may rain down
as programmed. Fortunately, we never had a real fire. Only charred
toaster tarts or something similar setting off a smoke alarm in a
room. This was handled quickly and without the activation of the
whole fire warning system.

Early on, I had my first system-wide warning experience. The
intercom blasted at midnight "Fire has been detected in the building," repeat, repeat. "Please go to the nearest stairwell and exit the
building," repeat, repeat. At well over one hundred decibels, the
announcement continued, ad infinitum. I had been given no prior
verbal instructions nor had anyone else, it seemed, about procedures.
Would a CNA come? One did not. That first time around, I stayed
in my room. None the worse for wear. The second time a CNA
came and shooed us to the end of the hallway; wheelchairs, walkers,
and all to wait in front of the stairwell door. Then it was over. Two
self-theorized hypotheses by residents emerged from these episodes.
If we hear fire truck sirens, go to the stairwell. If not, we stay in our
rooms. The doors were supposedly fireproof. Whether or not this
was correct, we never knew.

Naivety in thinking we're impervious to disrespect or harm in
a care-giving facility led me to take on the super sleuth mode once
again. A frightening and incongruous event set me in motion. I can
now relate these occurrences without angst, but I was mortified
while they were happening. The new fiasco started while I was

peacefully resting on my bed around lunchtime. I smelled slightly acrid smoke coming into my room. A bit of renovation had been going on in the next-door apartment. Maybe someone had burnt some wiring. More and more smoke came out of the vent. Then it began to billow, setting off my smoke alarm. Quickly, I wheelchaired out the door and yelled to a CNA who was bringing around lunch. "I can't stay in there; it's full of smoke." She radioed someone.

Shortly, a rather new maintenance man came up, disabled the alarm, and opened the windows to air out the apartment. He knew a smoke bomb had gone off and was puzzled about why. He told me maintenance staff had not been alerted, or residents, as would be the usual case. The smoke alarm triggered no other alert systems but two or three other smoke alarms. They also had to be disabled when the smoke vented downward. After the fact, an intercom announcement told CNAs to bring residents to the first floor if they reported smelling smoke. Nothing about this event set well with me. Finally, what seemed to be a concocted story made the rounds using the same exact wording. Plumbers had set off a smoke bomb in the toiletry system in a fourth-floor apartment, two floors below me, to locate a clog. If that were true, is that how it should have been handled?

I called my former plumbing company and gave them an earful. "Is that how you would have managed a like situation in an AL facility?" I asked.

"Absolutely not!" they resoundingly replied.

They went on to reassure me that the acrid smoke was non-toxic, and they added that bombs do come in agreeable scents such as peppermint or lilac. I would have preferred the aroma of a baking cinnamon bun.

I called the Ombudsman again, telling my story to a volunteer. I suggested I was the target. I had seen an orange, industrial electrical cord running from my hallway's baseboard outlet into the stairwell door that accessed the attic space. The maintenance man noticed that I had noticed. The volunteer asked me whom I wanted her to call, and I said the ED. She did not call him. Instead, she called the AL director who by that time had been filled in with the concocted story. I was suspicious, and the volunteer knew it. However, I was now of no mind to continue pursuing it with her. After time had elapsed, I noticed our contracted plumbing company's truck in the parking lot and took down their phone number. I called about the shenanigans giving a three to four-day window of time when the bomb had gone off, although I did remember the day. She could find no smoke bomb entries. What was I to do but call the ED. I left word that the initiator of the action, knowing it was the facility manager, had committed a job-terminating type of offense. No reply. Nothing changed.

The Showdown

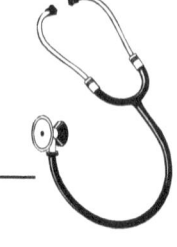

After experiencing five morally bereft transgressions with no acknowledgment by AL of wrongdoing, I knew it was time to send a projectile into the corporate arena. I wrote a meant-to-shock letter attaching supporting documents and mailed the packet of fourteen pages to the corporate president/CEO. Copies went to my district's State Representative and my attorney as well, to underscore my distress. So as not to raise suspicion that I was on the warpath, I had to handle the task surreptitiously. A young, caring activity leader working for the summer knew there were "goings-on" with me and consented to make three copies at a copy machine well away from prying eyes. In return, I wrote a letter of recommendation for her future employment. We were both pleased.

It didn't take long for corporate warpath activation. Word went out to the field director, to the executive director, and to me that a meeting would take place for the three of us. The only calls ever made to me by our ED were meeting related. On the first call, I asked if he had a copy of my grievances and he said yes, then intimated in a blustery tone that my complaints had no merit, and he would be the victor. Oh, the attitude. I couldn't fathom it coming from the head overseer of an elderly care facility in response to a resident seeking truth and accountability.

As happened, the meeting was postponed for a few days due to illness, not mine, but that of the field director. I was ready to get it over with. On the designated day, I wheelchaired into the ED's office. He and the field director were amid a conversation. I caught wind of the fact that he had not perused my letter until just that morning, not previously as stated. He'd been briefed, I'm sure, but without specifics. Now he was off guard and unprepared to fully discuss my issues. After an introduction to the field director, I too, became off guard when she bluntly asked, "What do you want?" I wish I had yelled, "Just have these miscreants fired!" But I knew she had a viable question and wanted to cut to the chase. I had signed a no litigation agreement as did all residents when entering this utopian care facility. Was I going to be asking to have an arbitration and be making a time-wasting stink?

Our discussion centered on manager involved infractions only. Small and devious Medicare fraud cases happen where there are small and devious people, no matter who's umbrella they're working under. First up came the incident of infestation. No official report had come from the pest control company's entomology lab showing result status. My question again was, "What happened to the specimen boxes?" The ED said he would check on it.

Then he asked ME, "What happened to the bag of dust?" How should I know, I thought. Probably disposed of just like the boxes. Leave no trace. My interest in a lab report was partly to avoid self-debasement. I knew there had been an insect egg case stuck on my lip. Not that it was relative to the lice infestation. It was not a hallucination, and I had put it in the specimen box. I wanted confirmation that I was not delusional and needed findings from the lab.

The second issue concerned the smoke bomb. After thorough sleuthing, I knew it was meant for me. If not, why wasn't a memo sent to residents about an upcoming maintenance procedure to fix a plumbing problem giving date, time, reassurance of safety, etc. I voiced my question, and the field director volleyed it to the ED with a perplexed facial expression. He became flustered, paged through his computer files to find a memo he thought had been written, but no luck. Then the field director gave the prompt to move on.

The third misdeed has yet to be mentioned but was included in my complaint to the corporation. On a Saturday when lower food chain managers take on ED duty giving the top one's weekend time, I had an unexpected visit from the on-duty manager. I was resting on my bed and heard a wee knock on my door. The facility manager entered saying, "I'm here to fix your TV." From the bedroom I replied that my TV was not broken, and I had not put in a maintenance request. Thinking he would just exit saying a mistake had been made with a sorry to follow, he did not.

I knew he had played with my two remotes messing up the signaling sequence I used for my TV. He then said, "I'll be right back," as though he needed to check on something TV related. He came back. A few minutes later he again said he would be right back. I wheelchaired to my entrance door and locked it. Another manager was covering the main office phones during lunch. I called to tell her about my dilemma and said I didn't want him in my room. Her reply, "You'll be lucky." When the field director heard this, she turned to the ED and said something to the effect that managers shouldn't be dissing other managers. That was her focus. There was no dismay over my feelings of intimidation. A little ruffling of the feathers never hurt anybody, right? As well as a little bullying. There was no record of a maintenance report. There was no broken TV.

Then the meeting was over at my request. I was tired. I no longer wished to remain in AL and said so. Perhaps by moving to independent living, I could leave those debasing events behind. I was told follow-ups would be made concerning my questions and complaints, and I would hear back.

Within Reason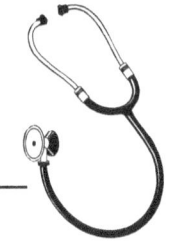

While my deepest wish was to leave corporate face-saving, heavy handedness behind, I wasn't going to force it into reality. Another housing do-over would have been a daunting task requiring family help with its accompanying mental and physical strain. So, I opted to move across the pond to the other side of the U-shaped campus, home to independent living residents. When I left the showdown meeting, I made a comment to the field director that I thought assisted living facilities should not be publicly traded corporate facilities. She looked at me quizzically and asked why. I told her the focus was on money, expansion, and higher salaried top managers. I wish I had added that the elderly and disabled are not commodities.

A few weeks after the showdown, the ED and his newly appointed assistant, having replaced my suspected Medicare fraud schemer, came to the activity room to fetch me for a meeting. We exited and went to the empty dining hall. First, the ED apologized for all I had gone through. He did not make denials and stated he would deal with the perpetrator, meaning the facility manager, in an appropriate manner.

I told him I felt like I'd been thrown under a truck, meaning bus, but the word eluded me. He said he felt the same way. I understood. The ED had no prior management experience for an entire care community. He had relied on steering from his machismo workmate. Soon, a very short memo went out saying the facility manager was no longer employed at the facility, and a search was underway for a replacement.

We continued the meeting. Then he said, "I have the reports

here." Not knowing what he meant, I questioned, "Reports?" Oh yes, the entomology reports from the contracted company's pest control lab. There was no report of any submission or examination of specimen boxes that had been retrieved from my apartment. The ED asked if there was anything else I wanted to know. I didn't want to rattle the cage any longer, so I said no. I was then offered payment to be moved to independent living. Everything would be taken care of. The movers would take pictures of my apartment so they could replicate furniture placement. I was still out-of-pocket for the parasitic, blood poacher treatment. I knew that was a lost cause.

There is seldom certainty of the reason why someone dislikes you and wants to maliciously harass you. Perhaps I looked like someone who had hurt him way back when. I had written a note or two about slap-dash painting and poor landscaping work by the contractors he had hired. They went into a locked box. I was voicing residents' comments as well as my own. Did he suspect I was the perpetrator? I did squawk loudly and repeatedly about having no protocol for my report of infestation and the complete disregard of my welfare. Lice lassitude, I labeled it.

I had to laugh about facility surveys. We were begged, I mean literally begged by top managers, to complete them. And I'm sure our managers were outright demanded by the corporate entity to get the task done. Out of four surveys conducted while I was there, only one came back with findings, and no beneficial changes ever took place.

If I could tamp down my negative remembrances of assisted living, I would do so. I doubt it will ever happen. I sensed a pervasive, uptight disunity shortly after taking up residence there. Later, I attributed poor functioning to unreasoned business modalities intertwined like 16 tentacles on two octopi in a wrestling match – a definite disablement resulting in no maneuvering ability and loss of direction.

Once I left AL, I considered my entire odyssey over. It can

evaporate to the nether world. Now it was time to reflect. I became intensely aware of human failure in my years of runaway decision making. We are endowed with the ability to reason, our highest power. One fact about this power is that around half of our brain mass is dedicated to decision making and problem solving. Yet we are still poor at weighing options and deciding which are both feasible and doable. We fail at looking at the big picture and taking a stand. In fact, decision making is often irrational.

I strongly believe that fact finding is one of the most valuable endeavors for creating solutions. It could have benefitted me and will benefit others facing medical crises. This narrative was not meant to be prescriptive. I cannot advise you about how to choose doctors or facilities, what to do when things go wrong, or who to call for help. I have written this as a testimonial that healthcare can and does go wrong. Putting on a thinking cap to deal with it can "Do no harm." As a tagline, a local West Palm Beach television station says, "The more you know." An excellent mantra.

It is fortunate my cognitive ability remained functional, maybe even more so, as all brain injuries are different. And now, in the aftermath of my odyssey, of sepsis crossing into the path of an injured brain, I am different, too. This tale was put together piece by painstaking piece – perhaps for the benefit it may have for those who read it.

IV

A STORIED TALE

Skintillations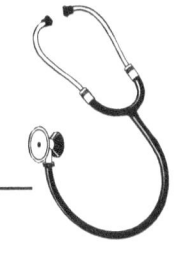

This added chapter highlights a quirky, odyssey-related adventure for the sake of levity. I had named the unknown oddity the White Dot Mystery. No one working in any medical capacity would comment about my strange skin condition. As I was making inroads investigating other unasked-for events, I decided to pacify myself by taking on this one as well. It satisfied my need-to-know passion, at least for a while.

The adventure centered around the largest and most complicated of our body organs, the skin. There might be as many as 3,000 skin disorders, and no sought-out dermatologist could give me a diagnosis of mine. Skin disturbances began during my hospital stay. I paid little attention. Then with a lice infestation prognosis and feeling skin-prickly, my focus began to change.

Resolution of whether I was lice infested was slow in coming. Attention was focused on the pandemic, and little regard for non-life-threatening complaints were given. Letter writing seemed to be my best option for illuminating the specifics of my situation. My communiques totally unendeared me to outreach entomologists with the University of Florida. Having limited address specifics, I generically sent two letters to their work locations. They ultimately reached the hands of the intended. I asked the entomology lab director for material from a textbook about lice. He phoned me, asked for a verbal description of my situation, then told me I absolutely did not have lice. Yet the lice had come, received sustenance, then went on their merry way. All at my expense.

Still, I felt something just under my skin. The second UF outreach entomologist had the term medical in her title. Could she enlighten me? What could it be but something else parasitic? We talked by phone about the especially unpleasing parasite, scabies. "You would know if you had them. You'd be on fire," she said. No, that wasn't the answer. I was not on fire.

Discouraged but pressing on, I sent her a few white dot samples. I had hoped that she might pass them on to some scientist with an all-encompassing curiosity like mine. I asked her to return the samples and email my daughter with any findings. The samples were not returned, and I believe they were discarded after receipt. However, my daughter did receive an email. The entomologist now became a turncoat. She had now become a psychiatrist and gave my daughter a recommendation that I may need an evaluation for delusional parasitosis. We were both appalled.

Extremely disgruntled at this point, I reviewed my need-to-know stance. But as a galvanized need to knower, I carried on the letter writing, albeit with risk of animosity. Missiles were sent to high profilers giving them skin descriptions, pictures, and dot samples. No one had business as usual during the pandemic. I'd projected their agendas were at a standstill, and they had become stymied. At least that thought mitigated my feeling of their disinterest. Perhaps the letters weren't received. Perhaps their screeners had nixed them. If by chance they were read, the letters didn't make the cut.

After making one last-ditch attempt for an answer, again fruitless, I moved my goal to one of surrounding myself with pleasantry. Need to know would be relegated to the second tier.

UPDATE: Many months later, a word I had seen on the internet by chance, crystalline, was the beginning of the mystery's unraveling. The name for my lumpy, rough and crusty skin, along with its prickly, stabbing sensations, would soon become known. Who would be the task master to find it? Why me, of course! The very same person who had diagnosed my trauma-related maladies over the past years when higher doctor gods could not. I will give credit, though, to those doctors who wrote journal articles and reports during the pandemic. This material ultimately appeared online and added to my skimpy data arsenal on skin conditions.

Crystalline was the spark that sent me flying through words, meanings, and concepts on the internet. One simple thought emerged. Crystal: hard and sharp with pokey edges, sounding like whatever was just under my skin. Salt crystals, metals, diamonds, and snowflakes are examples of crystalline substances. Pushing on with my science foray, I found my skin was infused with the alkaline Earth metal, calcium. It comes from the stars. Did I now feel like a starlet? Not on your life! Someone, take it away! In my teeth, my bones, but please not under my skin.

The condition is called calcinosis cutis. It is said to be rare and sometimes associated with other diseases, none of which I have. Online data led me to believe mine originated from the sepsis trauma.

Dermatologists had given me various remarks when examining my hands. One said, "Nothing can be done about the lumps," although no diagnosis was given. "Don't scrape at it," I was admonished. Of course I did, using the greatest microdermabrasion tool ever, the edge of a fingernail. I was told by a participant in my writer's group that his dermatologist referred to it as fingernail surgery. Along with those remarks came the psychological spiel. Time spent scraping was robbing me of participating in more meaningful activities. Yes? Like missing the Over Eighties Rock Group's performance at my independent living facility? I'd rather play scientist. Another doctor's comment after remarking I thought blood vessels were involved was, "No, it doesn't work like that." I'm satisfied now with my own skin diagnosis as confirmed by my new primary care physician.

While I'm no longer automatically thinking of situational song lyrics, I did find one lyric which suits this now-solved mystery. In my case, the song's sentiment is not meant for describing a relationship with an attractive, well-aged companion. Instead, it sums up one more of my unusual odyssey's state of affairs with the lyrical lamentation, *"I've Got You Under My Skin,"* best sung in somber musical tones.

About the Author

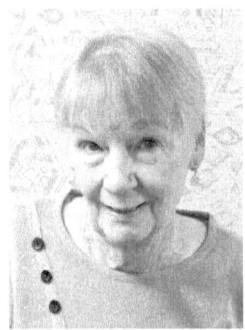

Who could write a more poignant account of a gone-wrong health-care tragedy than the patient? Her long history in public information writing for a renowned government agency qualifies her to succinctly reveal healthcare dysfunction as she experienced it. Her journey through a hospital, nursing home, and assisted living tells it all.

www.ingramcontent.com/pod-product-compliance
Lightning Source LLC
Chambersburg PA
CBHW021439210526
45463CB00002B/576